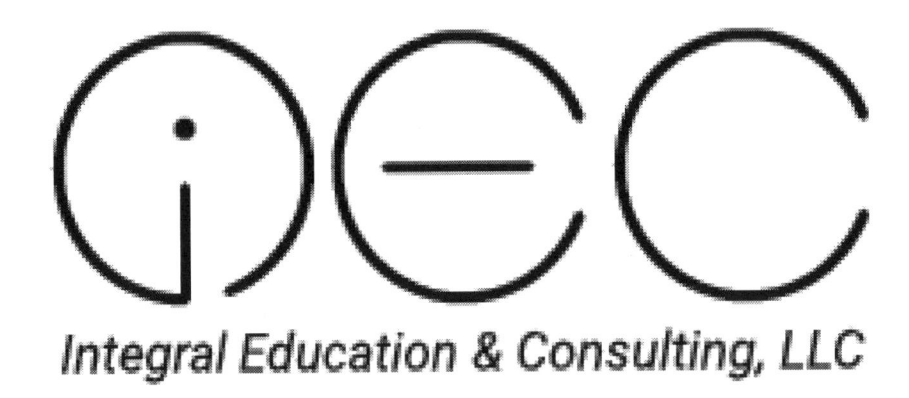

Cannacian™ Certification is a product of

iec

Integral Education & Consulting, LLC

Cannacian™ Level Three Certification

Presented in collaboration with

The eCS Therapy Center's Plant a Seed for Cannabis Eduation Tour

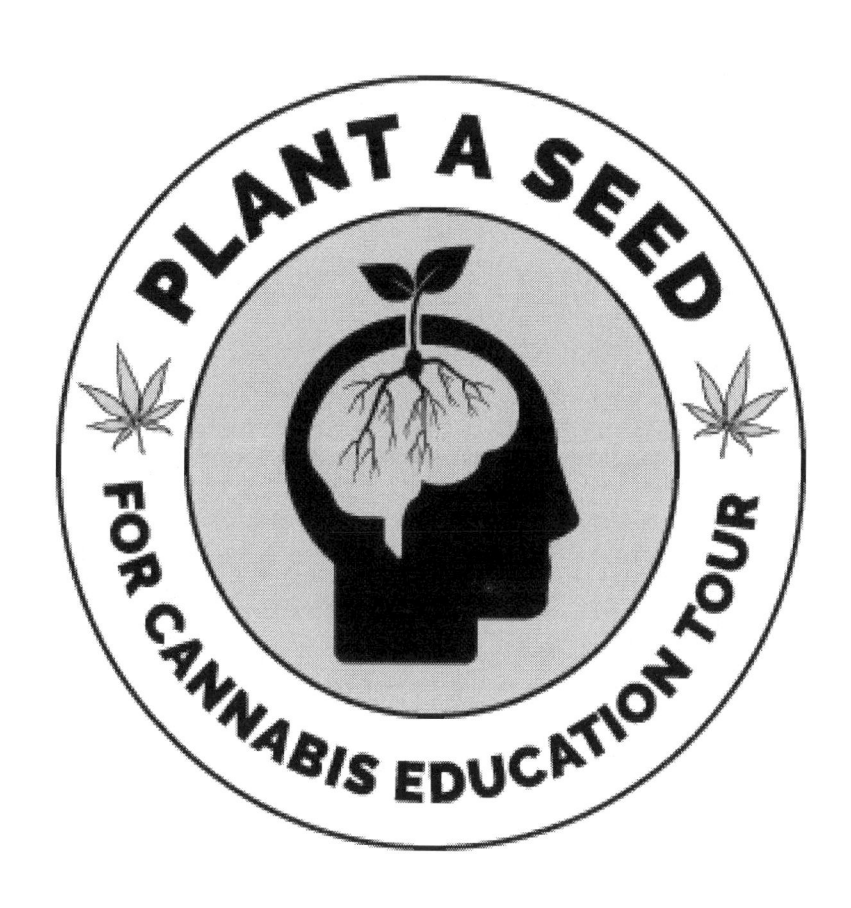

The Cannacian™ Level Three Training is offered by The eCS Therapy Center, Dr. Regina Nelson and experienced Cannacian™ Level Three Trainers. Classes have been accredited for Continuing Medical Education (C.M.E.) and other accreditng boards for continuing education credit, and is offered to the public as Cannacian™ Level Three Certification. All curriculum has been written and copyrighted by Dr. Regina Nelson.

Dr. Nelson is not a medical professional but has earned a Ph.D. in Ethical and Creative Leadership. She is an educational leader in the cannabis industry and medical cannabis patient.

If you are interested in becoming a Cannacian™ Trainer email a cover letter and CV to Regina@MyECSTherapy.org An investment in Training is required.
www.IntegralEducationandConsulting.com
www.myecstherapy.org

IISBN: 9781691691173
Imprint: Independently published by Integral Education & Consulting, LLC
Content/Graphic Support: Tab Moura

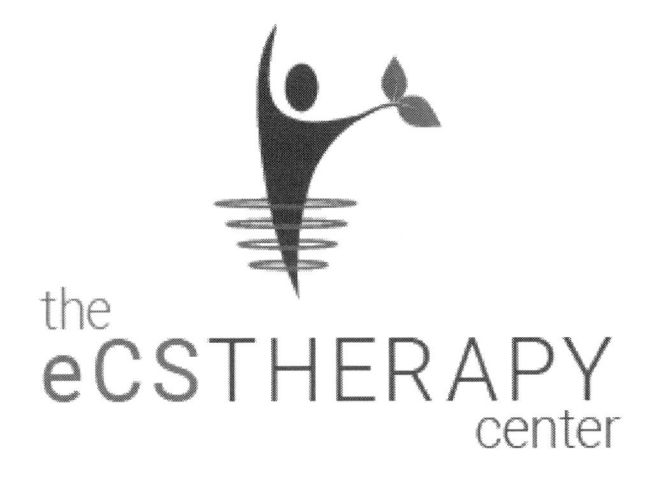

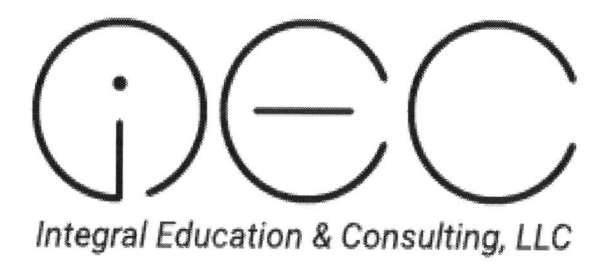

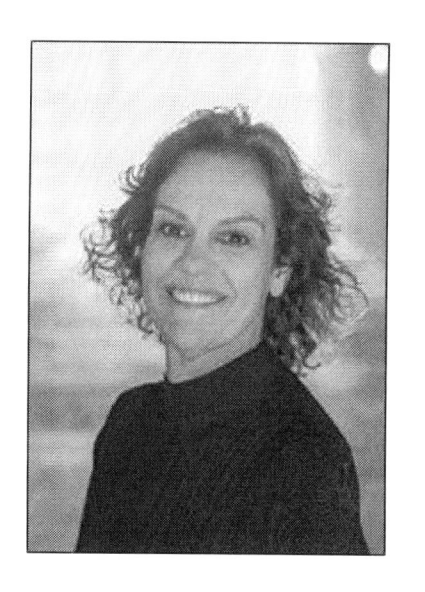

DR. REGINA NELSON earned her Ph.D. in Ethical and Creative Leadership at Union Institute and University in 2016. Her doctoral studies concentrated on Medical Cannabis. She has been publishing peer-reviewed articles since 2012, engaged in national cannabis education since 2013, and began presenting topical research projects in 2015. Nelson is a well-recognized public speaker in leadership, public policy, Integral theory, public health, and cannabis arenas. She is also the author of multiple titles including: *Theorist-at-Large: One Woman's Ambiguous Journey into Medical Cannabis*, *The Medical Cannabis Recommendation: An Integral Exploration of Doctor-Patient Experiences*, *Time for the Talk: Talking to Your Doctor or Patient about Medical Cannabis* and *The Survivor's Guide to Medical Cannabis*.

Dr. Nelson is a Founding Officer and current President of The eCS Therapy Center a 501(c)(3) Integral organization and national champion of community-based education and research projects.

www.myecstherapy.org

She also leads Integral Education & Consulting, LLC as C.E.O. providing cannabis consulting services, private education for organizational groups, and leading research projects for cannabis organizations.

www.IntegralEducationandConsulting.com

Much of the information regarding the endocannabinoid system (eCS) or the use of cannabis as medicine are referenced from Dr. Nelson's book, *The Survivor's Guide to Medical Cannabis*.

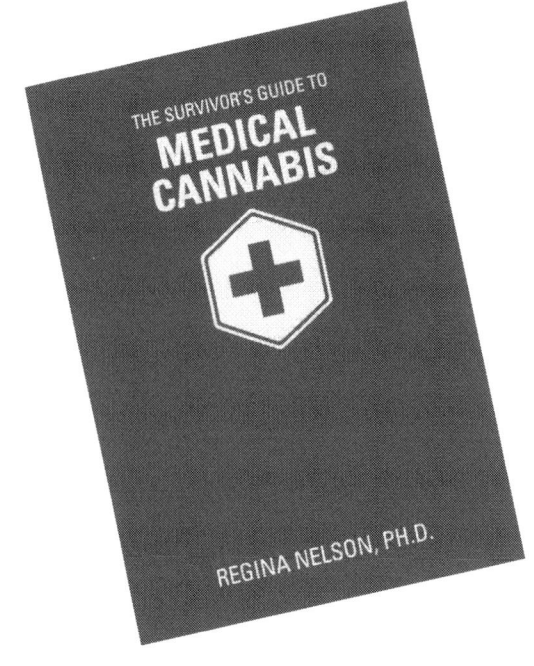

Join a Team of Cannacian™ Certified Trainers

Cannacian™ Certified Trainers are required to attend an online Train-the-Trainer Sessions for each Level of Certification. The training session includes a one-on-one session with Dr. Nelson. For more information email Regina@myecstherapy.org or visit www.myecstherapy.org for our next scheduled Trainer events.

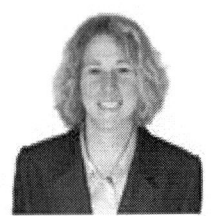

Tiffany Stuhr
Educator and Patient Advisor

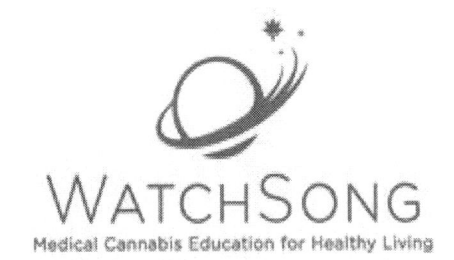

WATCHSONG
Medical Cannabis Education for Healthy Living

Cannacian™ Training Gave Me Back My Life

For ten years, I was broken. Chronic back and pelvic pain kept me dependent on opioids. The only western medicine answer was to keep taking them for the rest of my life. I had no idea how dull, lifeless, and devoid life had become. Then, I discovered medical cannabis. My journey with medical cannabis was rocky, full of trial and error, and wasted precious time and money. I ultimately transformed pain and misery into a passion for educating other medical cannabis patients and industry professionals.

Two years ago CBD oil was gaining popularity as a tool to treat opioid withdrawal. It wasn't easy, but I used it to wean off opioids. CBD alone did not effectively manage my pain and I turned to THC-based products. I had many uncomfortable experiences experimenting with strains, terpenes, consumption methods, and dosing. Nothing was straightforward and I set out to fill my knowledge gap with every bit of information I could find. Then, Dr. Regina Nelson, PhD with ECS Therapy Center entered my life.

I jumped at the chance to learn from an expert, since so few offerings seemed as rich in content on the subject, nor had accreditation provided by an experienced academic. I was blown away, not only by the depth of information, but by the insight into how I could apply the training to my own therapy planning. I walked away completely excited to...

- Know the physiological reasons why cannabis works
- Understand why it's so important to consider health conditions and medications while using cannabis
- Spot quality vs. sub-par products
- Out of all the available products and consumption methods, know which might be best suited for me
- Dose comfortably and safely to achieve maximum therapeutic effect

The Result? Today, I am opioid-free and in significantly less pain. I know joy that I've never felt, walk my dogs, swim, eat a vegan diet and lost 50 pounds. I've rekindled amazing relationships with friends and family. I wake up feeling refreshed and ready to approach life with vigor and excitement. The best part...

I created Watchsong, Medical Cannabis Education for Healthy Living. I now serve patients and industry professionals in a way I couldn't serve myself two years ago, through straightforward education that creates relief and revitalization. I am a trusted patient advisor that crafts hands-on, completely customized, unlimited support, medical cannabis therapy programs. To the patient-focused dispensary, I help position them to become experts in the community, increase sales, and step up from their competition. For doctors and clinics, I am a complete educational resource for patients.

Medical cannabis therapy is not a one size, fits all solution.
Effective relief takes education, planning, commitment, and time.
Find your path and your freedom today!

www.WatchSong.net

Tiffany Stuhr has a Bachelor's of Science degree in Biology and holds medical cannabis teaching certifications for Cannacian™ Level One & Two, pending Level Three. She is a conference speaker and writes articles for industry publications.

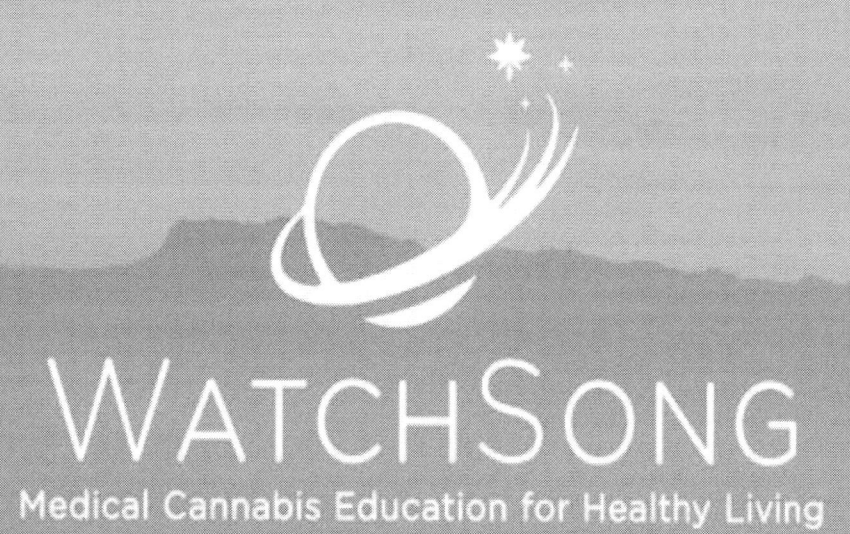

WATCHSONG
Medical Cannabis Education for Healthy Living

Learn How Patients are Reclaiming Their Lives Faster for Less Money

In this FREE webinar discover how you too can live with renewed purpose and freedom from debilitating pain, depression, anxiety and insomnia.

REGISTER FREE HERE > MJEducate.com

About Chef Tony & Green and Clean Chefs

Green and Clean Gourmet Chefs (G&C) began as an educational and private chef service to help people learn how to incorporate more infused plants into their nutritional plans. This is very personal to Chef Tony because he used Cannabis infused cooking to create customized healing protocols for his chronic pain and even depression/anxiety. The mission of G&C is to "Go Green and Get Clean." The truth is when people "Go Green" and get more plants their bodies will "Get Clean" but only if the plants are clean themselves; so we like to define clean as chemical free. The reality is so much of our food today is far from clean and if we want to optimize our bodies then it is time to eat cleaner (or chemical free). Our bodies are designed in such a way that we should all be considering our own Cannabinoid nutritional levels, which is part of what we help people discover at G&C led by Executive Chef Anthony G Freitas Sr. aka Chef Tony.

G&C is proud to offer private chef services for green and clean cooking classes, nutritional coaching, cooking events, and even private parties in your own home or business. Follow us on Facebook @GreenandCleanChefs for more information and look for Chef Tony at statewide events.

More About Chef Tony

Chef Tony has enjoyed a life filled with a wide range of diverse life experiences. Growing up as child in California, Colorado, and Oklahoma he saw life from a completely different perspective during his high school years living abroad in Brazil. With a family heritage that includes Portuguese and Greek descendants it only spurred his passion for culture, travel, and food from all over the world. His culinary arts interest started at the age of 5 when his Okie Gram started showing him how to help out in the kitchen for the holidays. From that age on he was always jumping at the chance to get into the kitchen and was incredibly blessed to learn not only from his Okie side but also his Greek Grandfather and always learning and helping his Mother, who is a world travelling and amazing home cook. The total now of 40 years of cooking experience was enhanced by working as a tableside flambé chef at a top Oklahoma country club. Utilizing these cooking skills and flavors from all over the world Chef Tony's new favorite skill is to infuse these international dishes with Cannabis Sativa.

Chef Tony has been cooking with Cannabis for almost 10 years now as a result of an automobile collision of a careless driver while riding a racing bicycle. This accident started an incredible journey, based upon culinary creativity paired with psychological research, in order to personally discover the healing properties of plants and the missing elements for nutritional healing. Through all this trial and error he is now passionate about sharing these experiences to help people find Green and Clean food in their lives for health and healing.

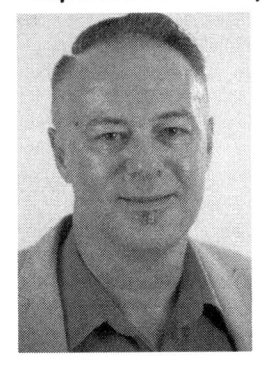

Chef Tony & The ECS Therapy Center

A healing story that includes nearly 10 years of cannabis research as a patient and a plant infusion chef reached a new pinnacle when Chef Tony received two Cannacian certifications from Dr. Regina Nelson. This education continued with a Cannacian trainer certification. The ECS Therapy Center and Dr. Nelson have expanded and supported Chef Tony's vision to serve people with forward thinking solutions about Cannabinoid Nutrition through education, coaching, and cleaner products.

CHEF TONY APPROVED

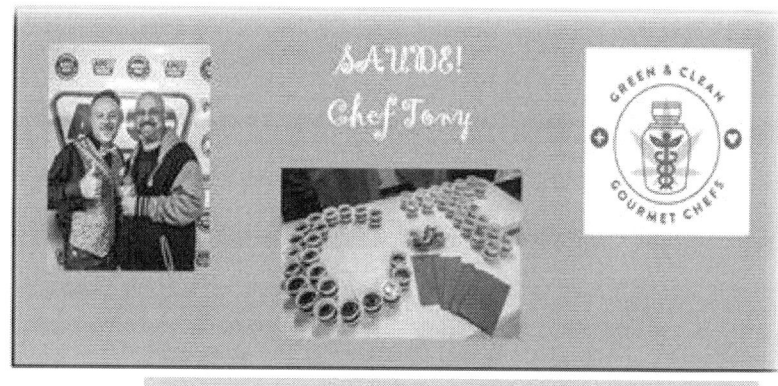

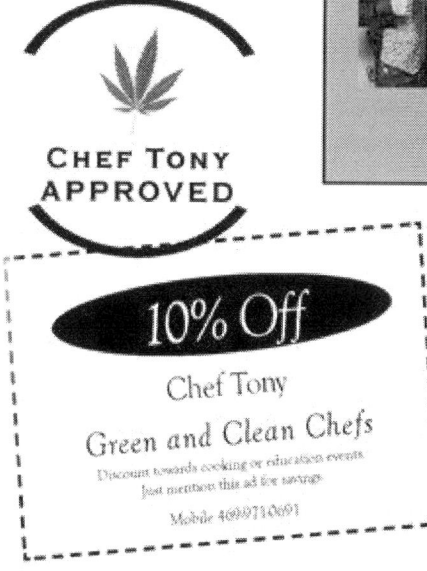

SAUDE! Chef Tony

GREEN & CLEAN GOURMET CHEFS

10% Off
Chef Tony
Green and Clean Chefs
Discount towards cooking or education events
Just mention this ad for savings
Mobile: 4699710691

Educational Topics

A multi-part curriculum for patients, caregivers, and commercial licensees to learn more about how to improve therapeutic benefits by treating Cannabis more as a food. This curriculum includes the following options:

- Cooking with Cannabinoids
- Cannabis as a SuperFood
- Customizing Healing Protocols
- Cannabis in Your Kitchen
- Cannacian Level 1 Training

Infused Diner Parties

Infusion dinners can be scheduled with Chef Tony as your very own in home private infusion chef. During these events, Chef Tony will work to custom infuse any Cannabis product provided. Currently, using all Oklahoma approved Hemp products for dinners. Other full spectrum items can be infused for OMMA card holders depending on host. All events include a team of culinary professionals, including other chefs, to provide an incredible gourmet 5 course meal and a unique culinary experience. Private parties can start for just 6 people in the privacy of the host's home for as little as $420. For all events we will work to customize the best solutions and provide private education about Cooking with Cannabinoids.

GREEN & CLEAN GOURMET CHEFS

Contact or Follow Chef Tony and Green and Clean Chefs through

Facebook: @GreenandCleanChefs
Instagram: @GreeenChefTony
Email: TFreitasOK@Gmail.com
Mobile: 469-971-0691

THE SURVIVOR'S GUIDE TO
MEDICAL CANNABIS

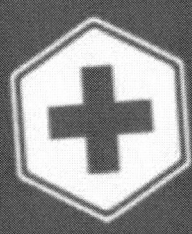

REGINA NELSON, PH.D.

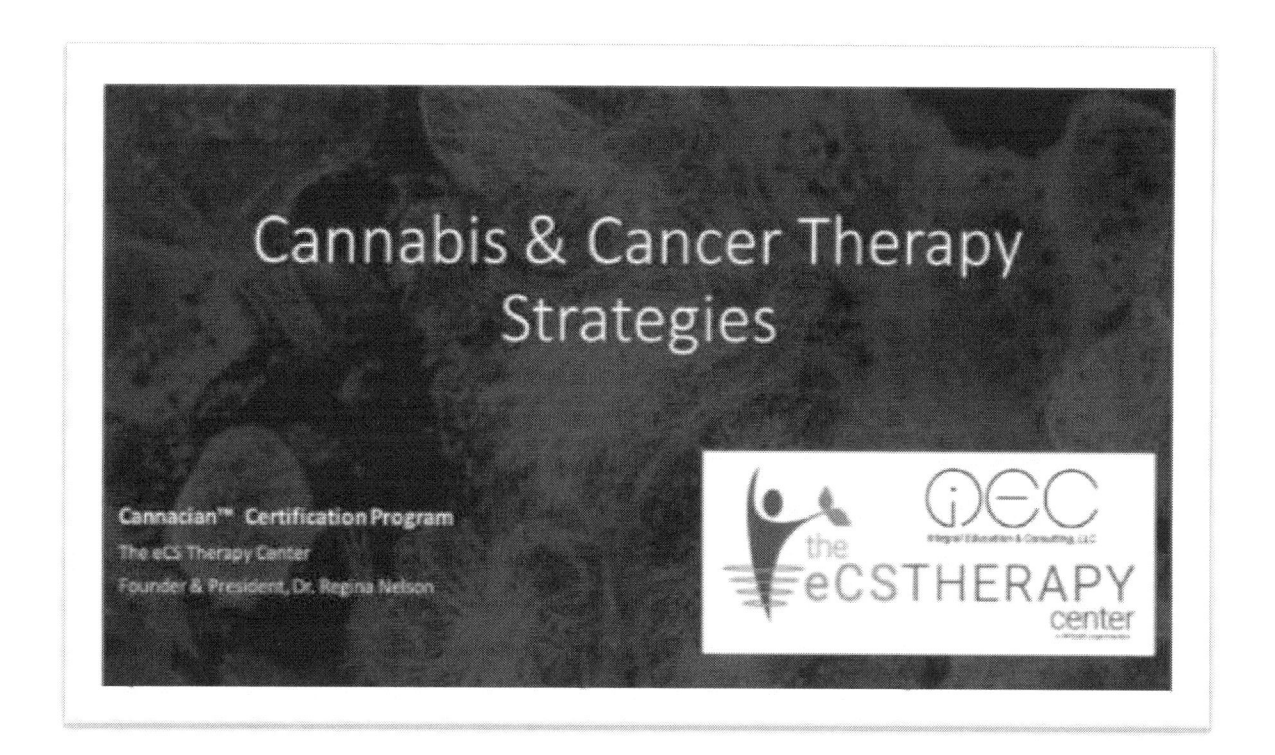

Welcome to Cannabis & Cancer Therapy Strategies. This is the second course in the Cannacian™ Level Three Certification program.

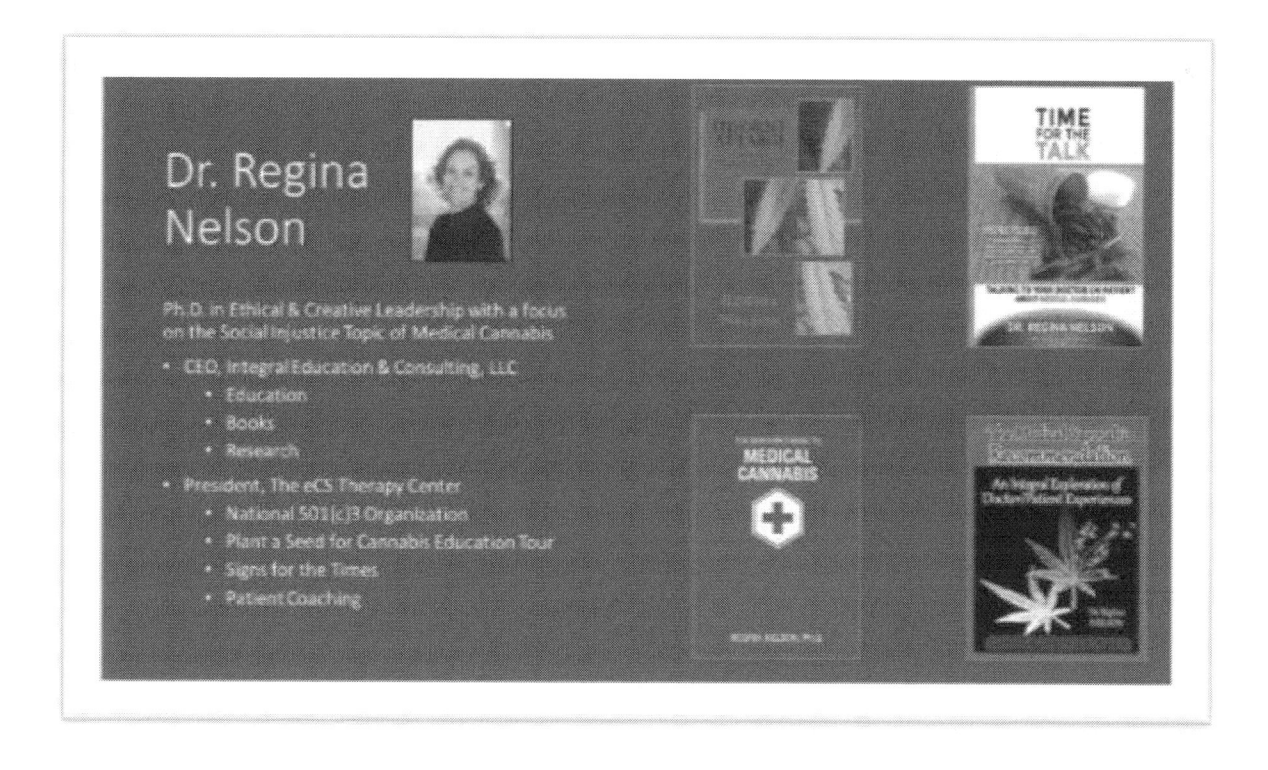

I am Dr. Regina Nelson, the author of this course. However, I am not a medical doctor, I am a Ph.D. in Ethical and Creative Leadership and I am a medical cannabis patient.

I began my journey into medical cannabis in 2010. Though I had been a long-time cannabis user, I'd become sick and I was looking for answers. Because I could find so little research, especial social research on the subject, I chose it as the topic to focus my degree in Ethics & Social Justice from Union Institute & University.

As a desperate patient in search of answers, I began attending the International Cannabinoid Research Society Symposiums in 2014, hoping that the greatest minds in cannabis science could help me understand how to use cannabis more effectively. I discovered two things during that first foray into science 1) the researchers most cited in cannabis know very little about how people use it and 2) animal studies point to therapeutic dosages in people. The year following that conference I began asking hundreds of patients how they use cannabis and how much they take—I came to find that people very clearly and naturally titrate their cannabis use to the animal study guidelines (especially when they are empowered to do so and having success)—or they won't--but those who do not, have much less success treating painful conditions without knowing how much cannabis might be helpful. I began sharing this information widely when I published "The eCS Therapy Companion Guide" in 2015. I republished this title in 2018, as *The Survivor's Guide to Medical Cannabis.*

The Cannacian™ Certification program was developed initially from *The Survivor's Guide to Medical Cannabis* but with the third and final module it has definitely grown beyond the book. The courses were developed as an "educated step-up" for not only bud-tenders, but others working in the cannabis industry. However, as the years have progressed and the curriculum has grown (and been accredited by multiple agencies), the audience seeking quality medical cannabis education has grown and we now see professionals from many industries seeking Cannacian™ certification for an educated step-up.

This third and final segment of the Cannacian™ Certification program has as a first session is "Cannabis & Cancer Therapy Planning Strategies." In this module we will discuss approaches medical cannabis patients consider when facing cancer. In the second module, "Cannabis Therapy Plans for the Chronically Ill," we will explore chronic illness and approaches to cannabis therapy throughout the life span. During the third module, "Cannabis and Opiate Withdrawal/Addiction," our discussion will focus on working with patients seeking to replace opiates with cannabis and/or other alternative therapies. And, finally, for the fourth and final module of the Cannacian™ Certification program our focus will be in "Cannabis & Seniors," as senior citizens are the fastest growing population of medical cannabis users.

I love to hear feedback from course participants, so please feel free to reach out to me via regina@myecstherapy.org. As well, educators seeking to take a career step-up and license the Cannacian™ Certification program should reach out as well. The Cannacian™ Training Network is expanding rapidly. Train-the-Trainer events are posted on myecstherapy.org.

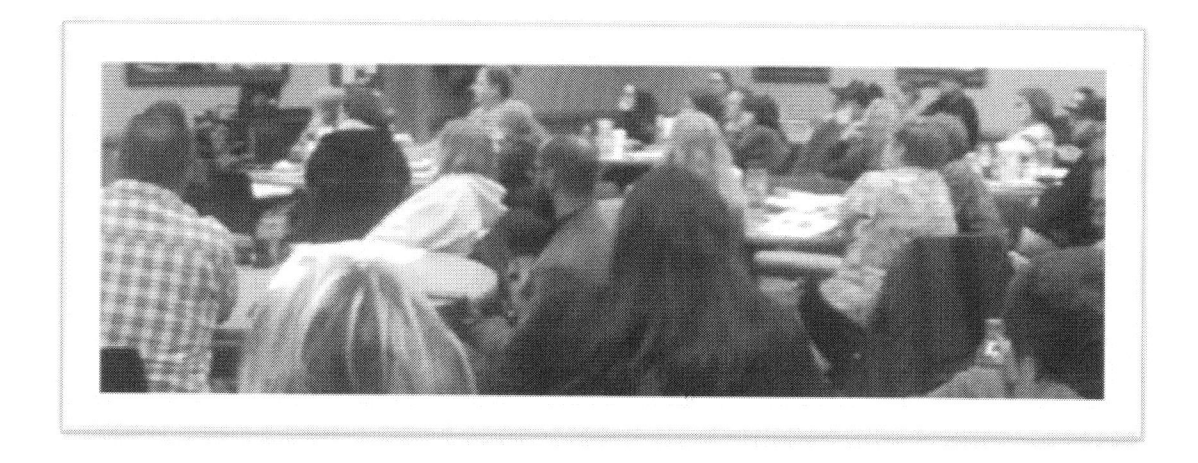

Best wishes,
Regina

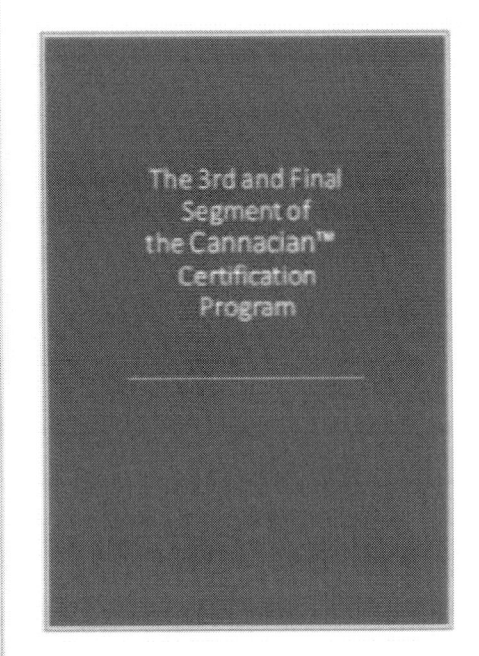

The 3rd and Final Segment of the Cannacian™ Certification Program

Cannacian™ Certification Courses

Regina Nelson, Ph.D.

Cannacian™ Level One Certification

Cannacian™ Level Two Certification

Cannacian™ Level Three Certification

Objectives

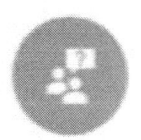

- DEFINE CANCER AND DISCUSS BOTH COMMON CONVENTIONAL AND ALTERNATIVE THERAPIES
- DISCUSS APPROACHES MEDICAL CANNABIS PATIENTS CONSIDER WHEN FACING CANCER
- CONSIDER CANNABIS COMMUNITY GUIDELINES VS. SCIENTIFIC EVIDENCE (ANIMAL STUDIES) WHEN APPROACHING CANCER WITH CANNABIS THERAPY
- DISCOVER THE DIFFERENCES BETWEEN SHORT AND LONG-TERM NEEDS OF CANCER PATIENTS SEEKING CANNABIS THERAPY OPTIONS

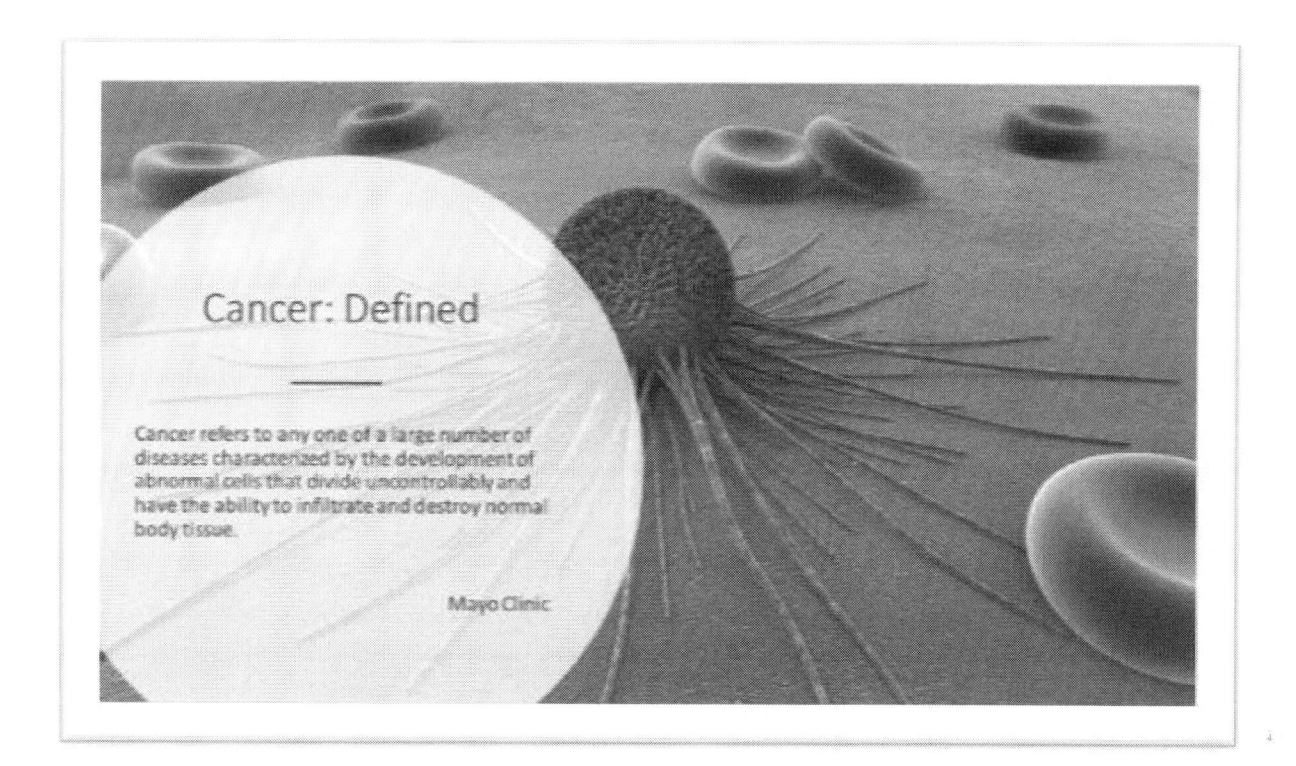

Cancer: Defined

Cancer refers to any one of a large number of diseases characterized by the development of abnormal cells that divide uncontrollably and have the ability to infiltrate and destroy normal body tissue.

Mayo Clinic

Cancer refers to any one of a large number of diseases characterized by the development of abnormal cells that divide uncontrollably and have the ability to infiltrate and destroy normal body tissue.
Cancer often has the ability to spread throughout your body.
Cancer is the second-leading cause of death in the world. one out of every two men, and well over one out of every three women in the US will develop cancer in their lifetime. This rate has risen to such an extent that cancer is now the leading cause of death in the US.

Notes

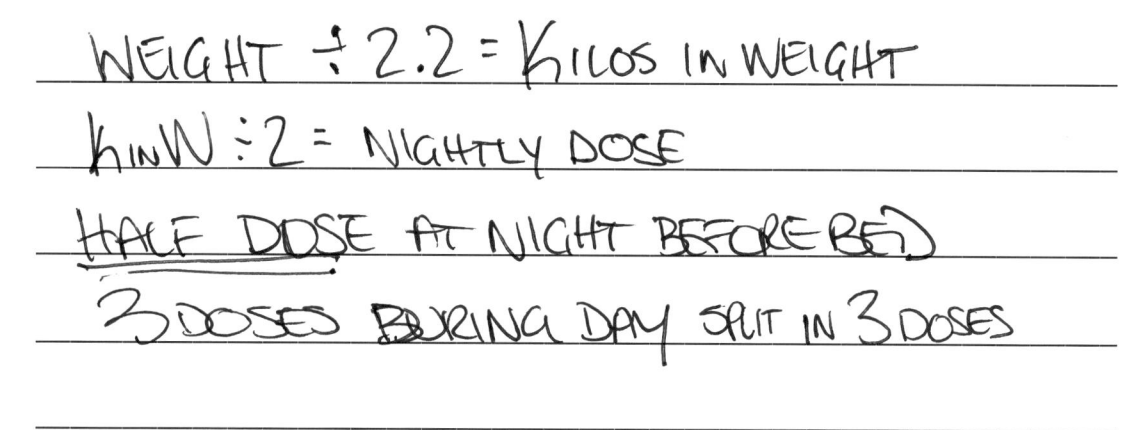

WEIGHT ÷ 2.2 = KILOS IN WEIGHT
KinW ÷ 2 = NIGHTLY DOSE
HALF DOSE AT NIGHT BEFORE BED
3 DOSES DURING DAY SPLIT IN 3 DOSES

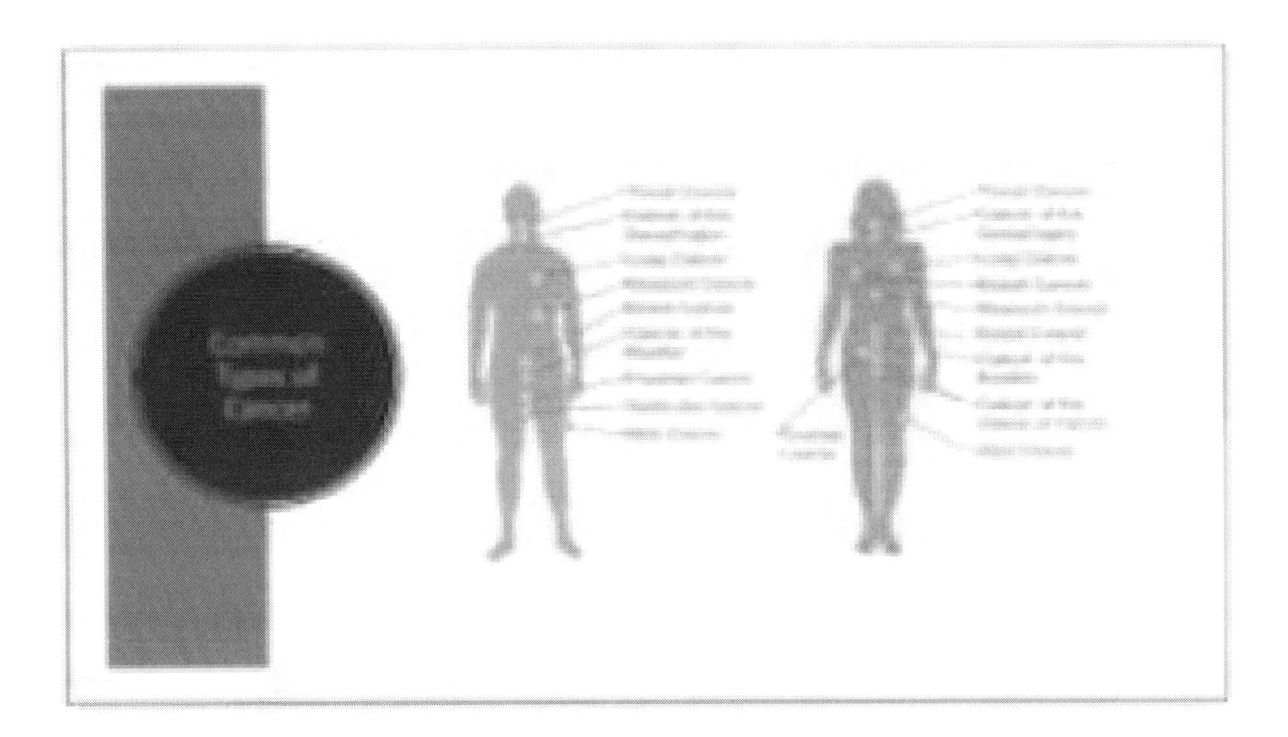

This list represents a list of only the most common forms of cancer. If you review information at the Cancer Society of America, you'll see there are literally hundreds of types of cancer..

Over the last several decades, as humans, we've violated our planet and spread cancer-causing agents that are not only in our air, soil, and water supplies, but also in our food.

Notes

- CHEMO WAS A BYPRODUCT OF WWII WARFARE
- CHEMO IS PSYTOTOXIC

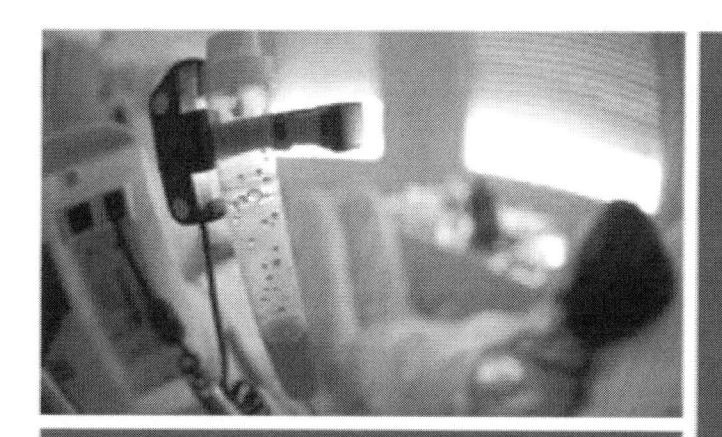

Conventional Cancer Approaches

conventional treatment
(kun-VEN-shuh-nul TREET-ment)
Treatment that is widely accepted and used by most healthcare professionals. It is different from alternative or complementary therapies, which are not as widely used. Examples of conventional treatment for cancer include chemotherapy, radiation therapy, and surgery. Also called conventional therapy.

Cancer.Gov

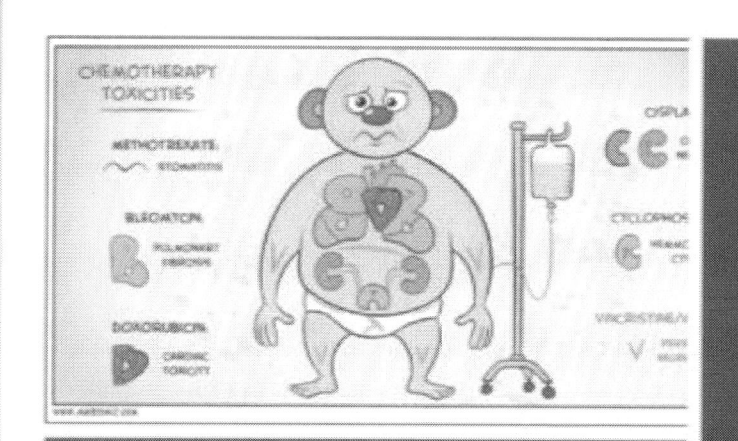

Common Side-Effects of Conventional Cancer Therapies

- Nausea & Vomiting
- Nerve Problems (Peripheral Neuropathy)
- Anemia   Appetite Loss
- Weight Loss   Pain   Fatigue
- Constipation/Diarrhea
- Bleeding/Bruising   Hair Loss
- Sleep Problems
- Skin & Nail Changes
- Sexual Health Issues
- Flu-Like Symptoms
- Urinary/Bladder Problems
- Mouth & Throat Issues
- Fertility Issues   Edema
- Various Infections or Organ-related Inflammation

Will an Oncologist Provide a Medical Cannabis Recommendation for a Patient?

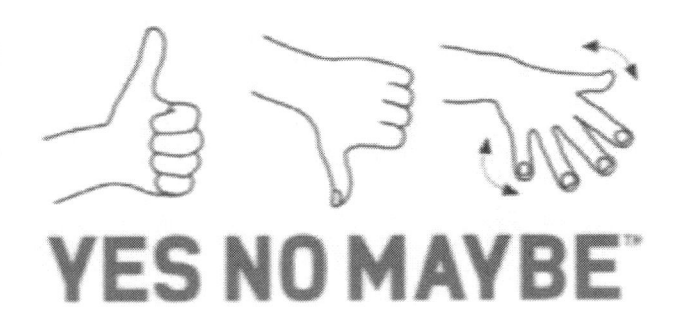

YES NO MAYBE

ONLY IF IT IS ALLOWED BY THEIR INSTITUTION

Alternative Approaches to Cancer

- Gerson Therapy
- Budwig Diet
- Proteolytic Enzyme Therapy (1906)
- Vitamin C Chelation (REMOVE CALCIUM DEPOSITS)
- Frankincense Therapy (Also Budwig)
- Probiotics (80% IMMUNE SYSTEM IN GUT)
- Sunshine & Vitamin D 3
- Turmeric and Curcumin
- Oxygen & Hyperbaric Chambers
- Prayer or Peace Building

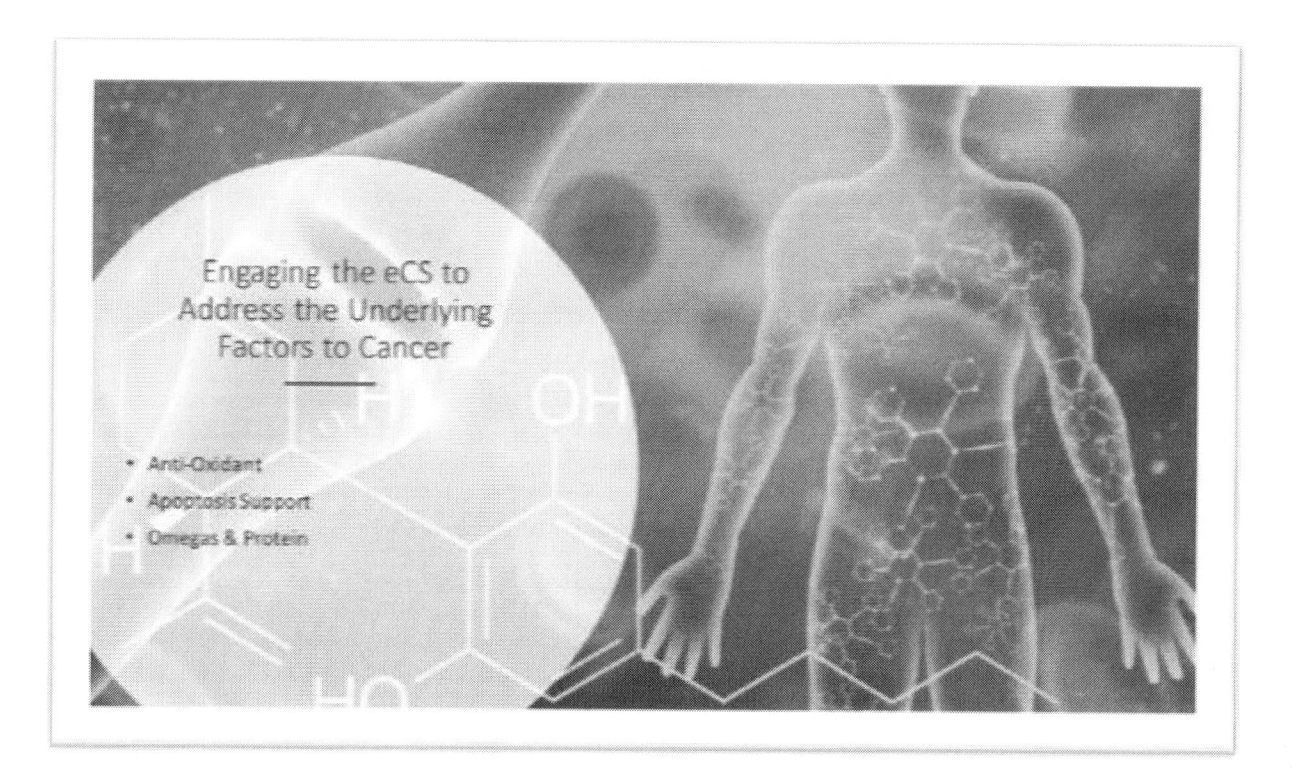

Engaging the eCS to Address the Underlying Factors to Cancer

- Anti-Oxidant
- Apoptosis Support
- Omegas & Protein

Anti-Oxidant: An **anti-oxidant** is a molecule that inhibits the oxidation of other molecules. Oxidation is a chemical reaction involving the loss of electrons or an increase in oxidation state. Oxidation reactions can produce free radicals. In turn, these radicals can start chain reactions. Antioxidants are found in many foods, including fruits and vegetables, including hemp seed and cannabis plants. In fact, CBD and THC have both been shown to be neuroprotective antioxidants.

Apoptosis Support: Cannabinoids in general, and specifically CBG, CBD, and THC have both been shown provide apoptosis support. Apoptosis is simply cellular death—and cannabinoids specifically target unhealthy cells, unlike chemotherapy.

Omegas & Protein: As an example, hemp protein powder contains 20 amino acids, 9 of which are essential amino acids that the human body can't produce on its own and needs from dietary sources. Healing via food is an old a philosophy as Socrates.

Patient Preference in Cannabis Therapy

- Feel Better and Treat Symptoms
- Hit it Hard like Canna-Chemo

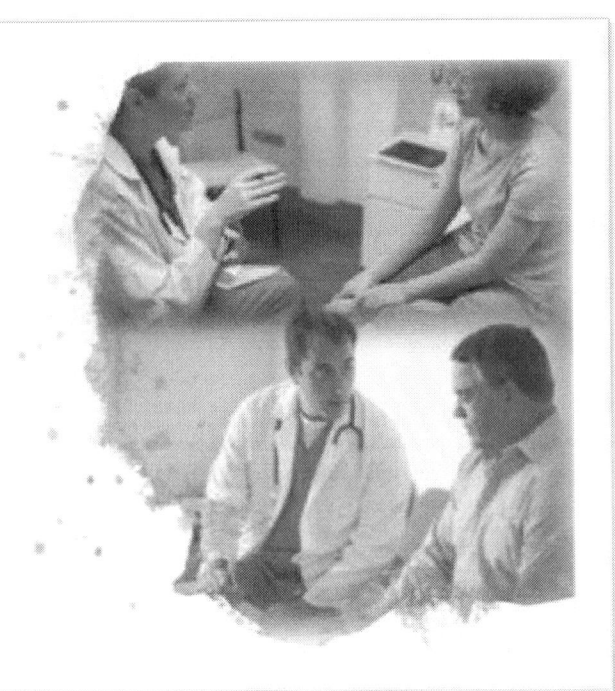

The two main appoaches to cancer therapy in the cannabis space are to treat to symptom relief (at least 1 mg per kilo) or to hit it hard like canna-chemo by titrating to very large doses of cannabis oil over a 90+ day period.

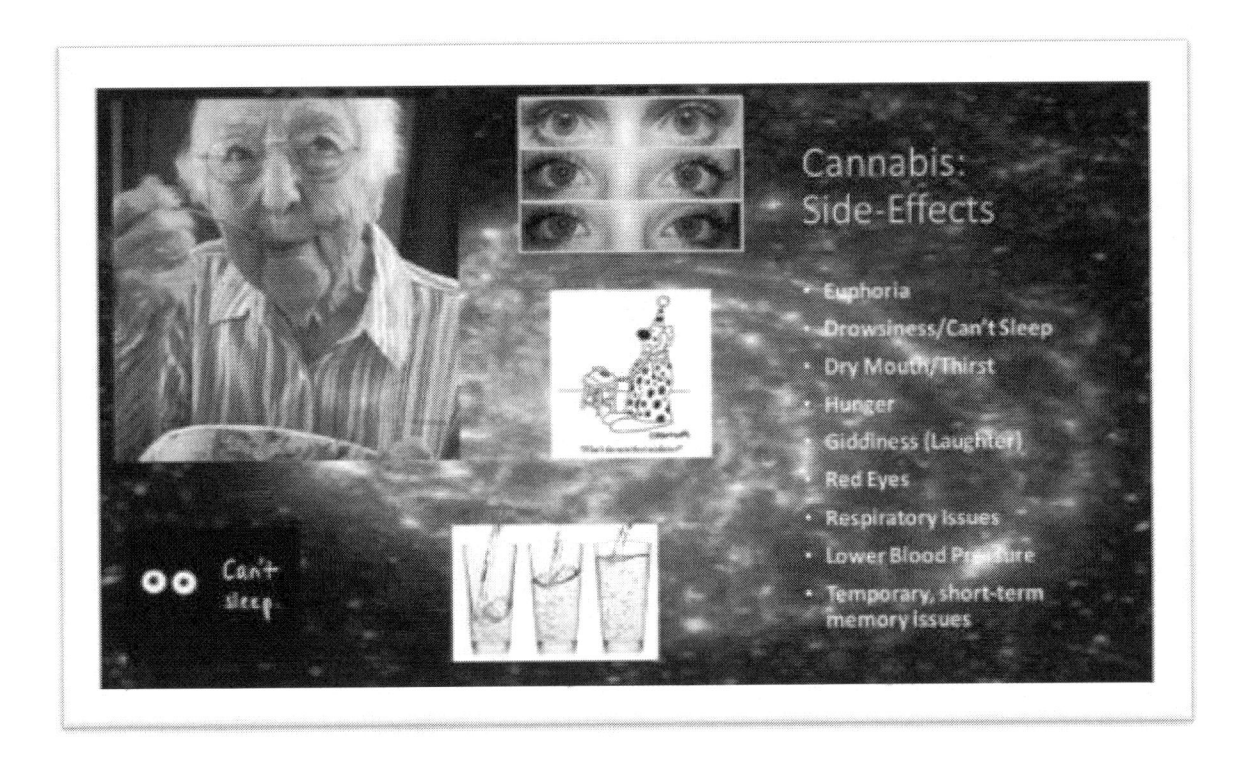

Cannabis: Side-Effects

- Euphoria
- Drowsiness/Can't Sleep
- Dry Mouth/Thirst
- Hunger
- Giddiness (Laughter)
- Red Eyes
- Respiratory Issues
- Lower Blood Pressure
- Temporary, short-term memory issues

The Euphoria Hurdle

- Broader Cannabinoid Profiles
- Raw/Fresh Cannabis
- THCa v. THC
- Addition of a Choline Supplement

Combining Cannabis with Conventional Cancer Therapies

- "Don't take with Grapefruit" Warnings—Heed them!
- Choline helps many patients titrate with cannabis oils, but choline should not be consumed by brain cancer or other cancer patients without discussion with the oncologist
- Begin cannabis therapy PRIOR to conventional treatments when possible
- It's never too late to add a cannabis supplement

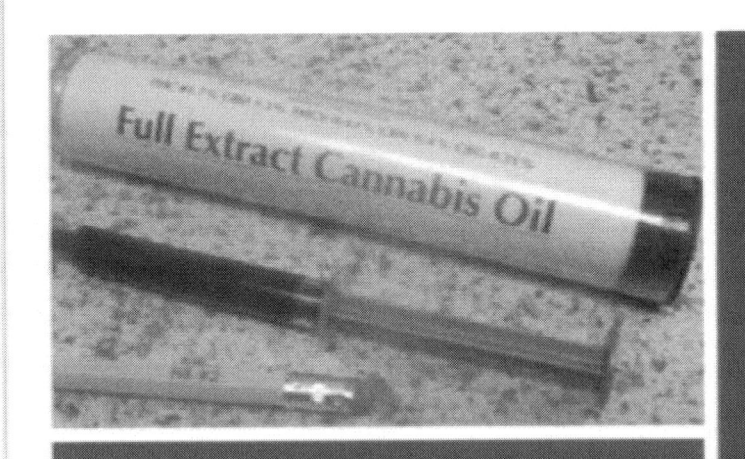

Cannabis Community Rule of Thumb

- 60 grams of cannabis oil in 90 days
- 30-45 day titration to 1 gram per day
- Titrating to 10 – 20 mg per kilo

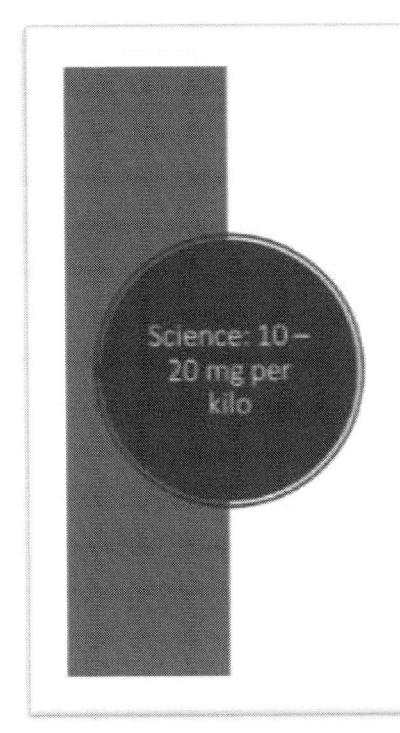

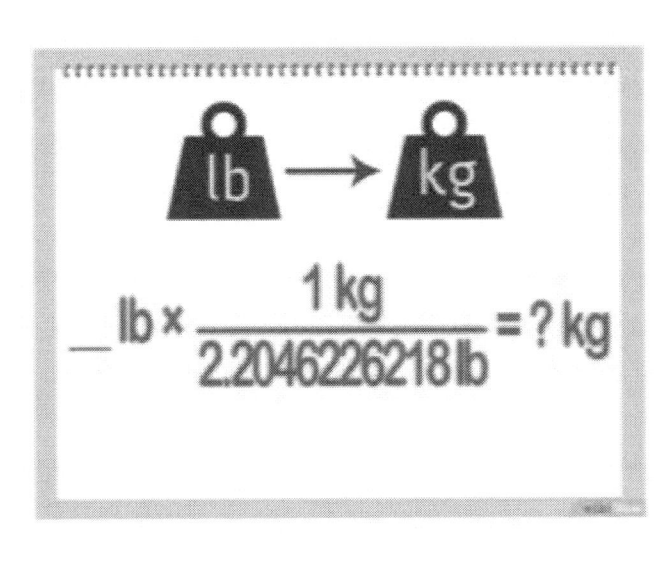

Science: 10 – 20 mg per kilo

$$\_\_ \text{lb} \times \frac{1 \text{ kg}}{2.2046226218 \text{ lb}} = ? \text{ kg}$$

Preferred Delivery Methods

Raw/Fresh Cannabis when possible

Cannabis Oil as a Base Medicine

Minimum Once per Day Edible Dose

Largest Dose of THC at Bedtime

Topical & Suppository added to Daily Regiment

Sublingual, Vapor or Smoke or Acute Relief of many Symptoms

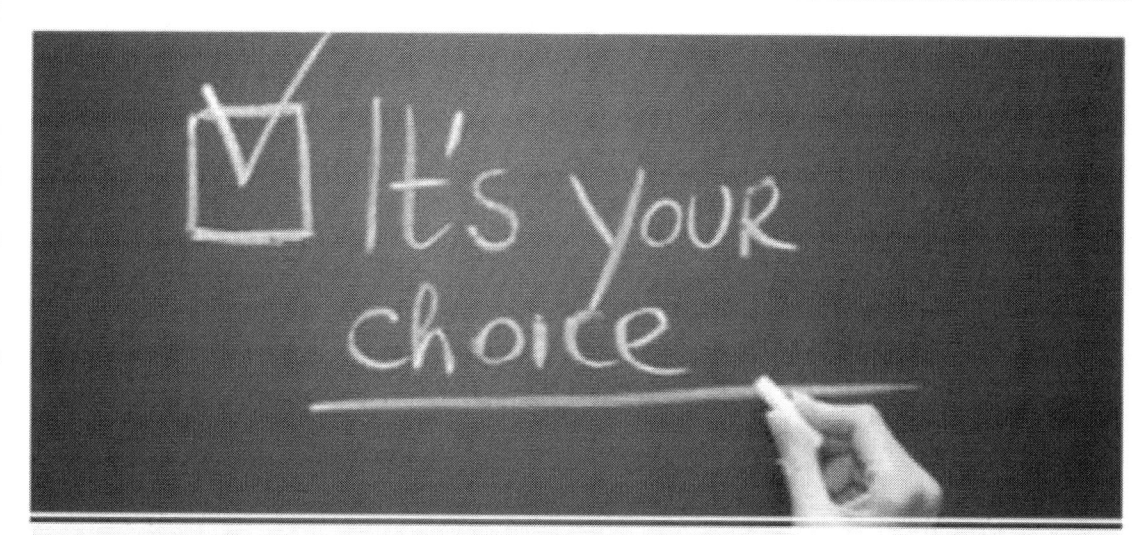

It's your choice

Cannabis Oil? Hemp Oil? or Both??

Dosing Differences based on Approach

Quality of Life
- Slowly titrate to 1 mg per kilo
- Continue titration slowly until the patient no longer wishes to increase the daily dose
- Maintain a steady and consistent daily dose

Hit it like Chemo
- Rapidly titrate to consuming 1000 mgs of cannabinoids per day
  - Some may wish to target 10 – 20 mg per kilo and titrate further
- Maintain 1000+mg of cannabis oil daily for 45 – 60 days
- Reduce dose to 5 mg per kilo as a daily dose

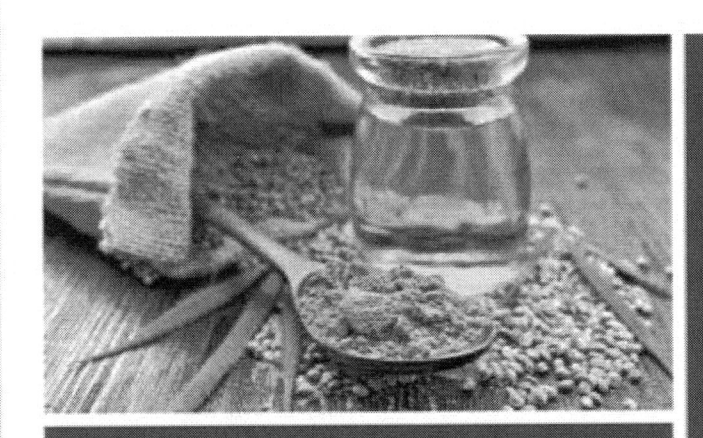

Long-Term Maintenance Dosing

- Suggested 2 – 5 mg per kilo
  - 2 – 5 years
- Minimum 1 mg per kilo
  - Life

Focus on Symptoms and Outcomes

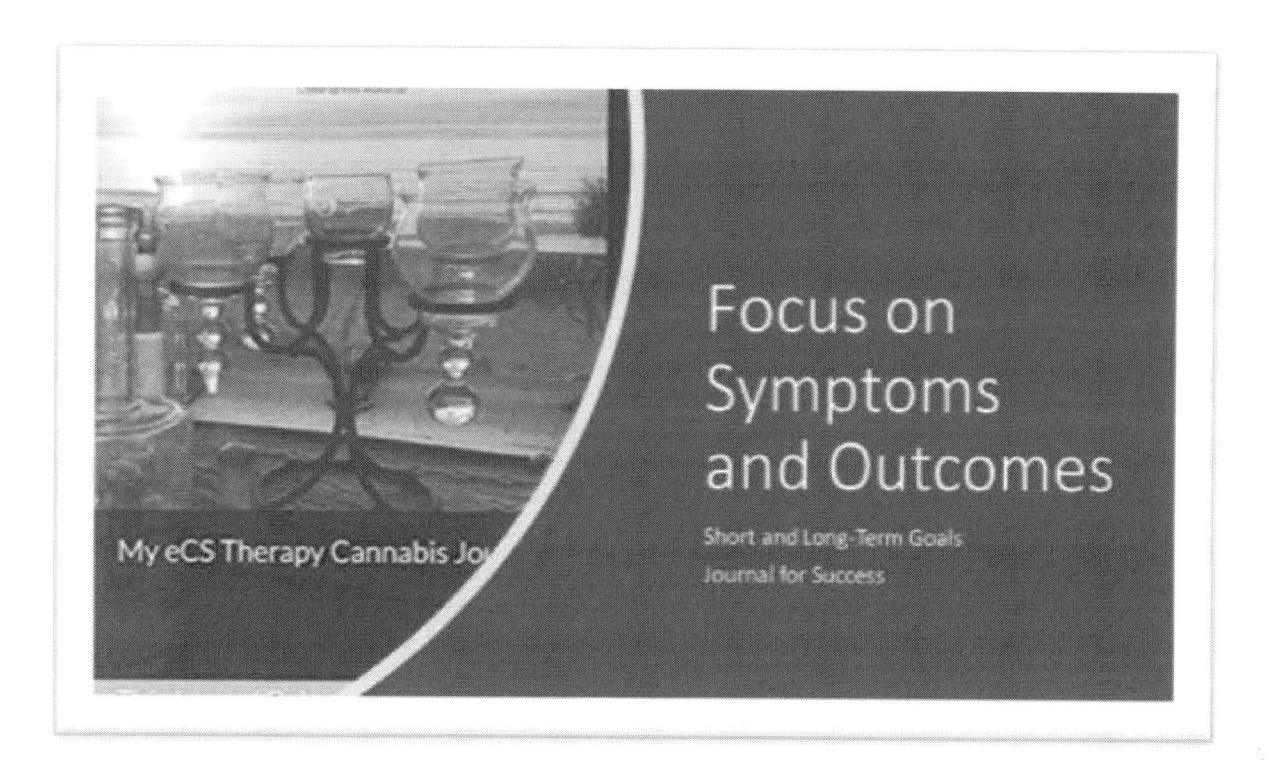

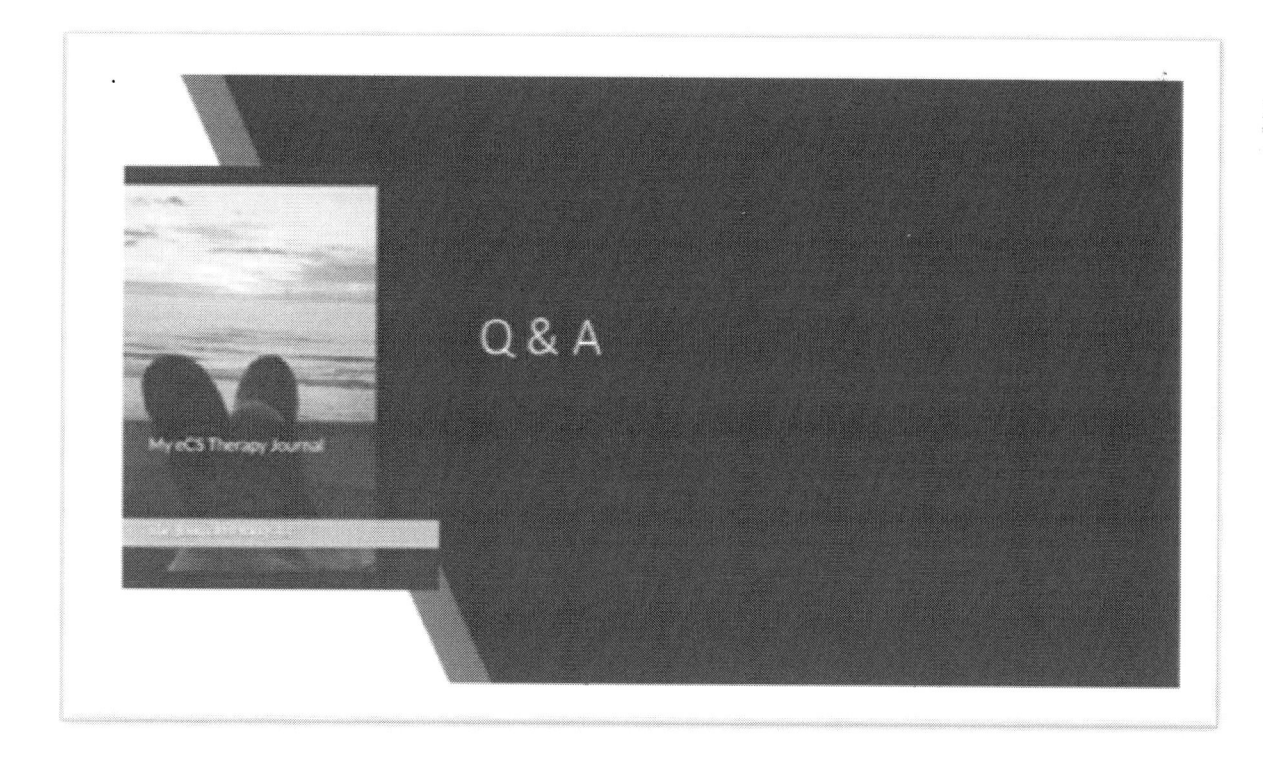

Short and Long-Term Goals
Journal for Success

My eCS Therapy Cannabis Journal

Q & A

My eCS Therapy Journal

Notes

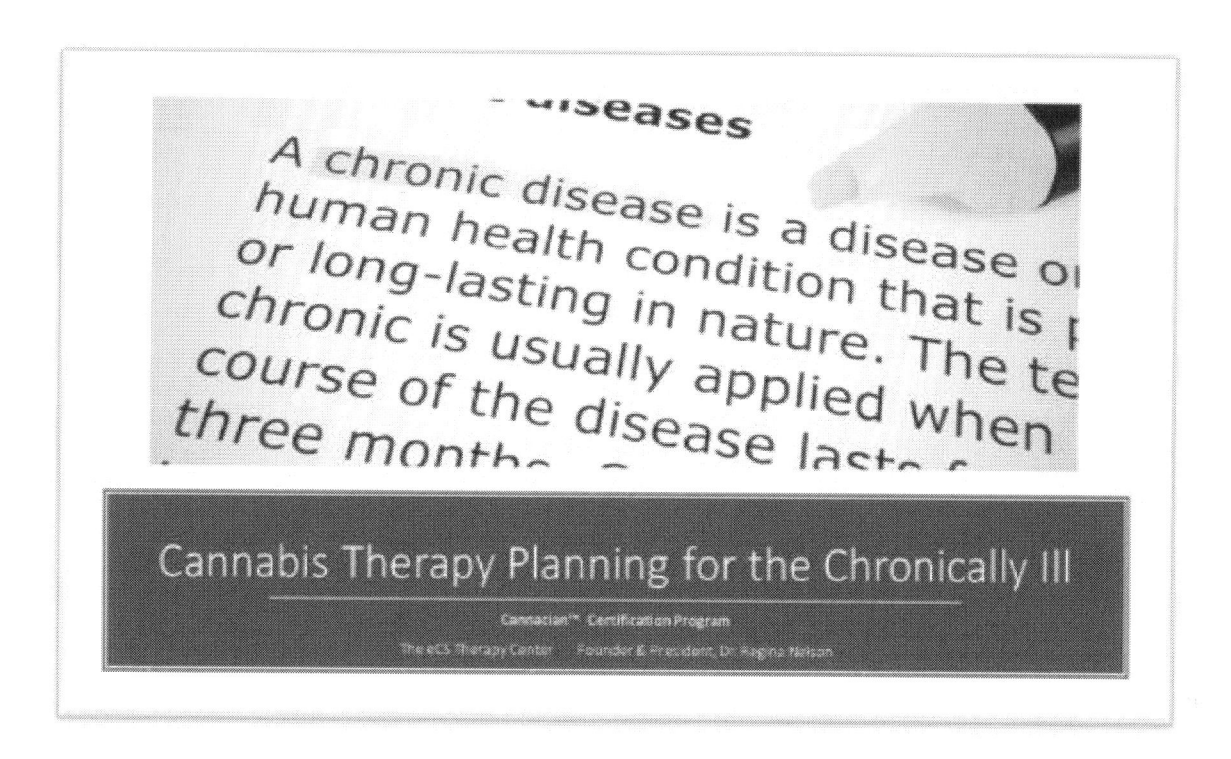

Cannabis Therapy Planning for the Chronically Ill

Cannacian™ Certification Program
The eCS Therapy Center Founder & President, Dr. Regina Nelson

Welcome to "Cannabis Therapy Planning for the Chronically Ill". This is the second module of the Cannacian™ Level Three Certification program.

Objectives

Define and Discover	Define and Discover what Chronic Illness is
Review	Review Common Chronic Illnesses
Discuss	Discuss the affects of Chronic Illness throughout Life Span
Review	Review Cannabis Dosing Guidelines
Explore	Explore Therapy Planning Techniques for Chronically Ill Medical Cannabis Patients

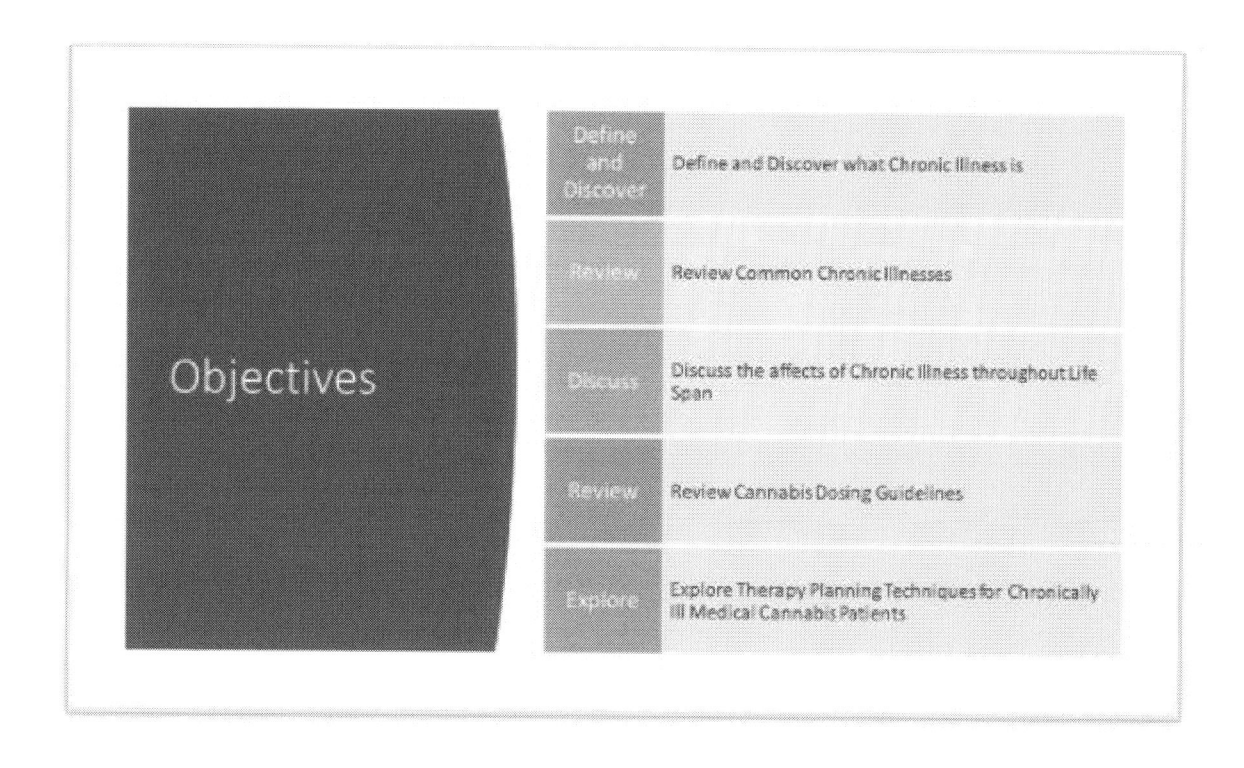

What does "Chronically ill" mean?

chronic illness
any disorder that persists over a long period and affects physical, emotional, intellectual, vocational, social, or spiritual functioning.

MORE THAN 50% OF THE WORLD LIVES WITH CHRONIC DISEASE

Most Common Chronic Illnesses in Children

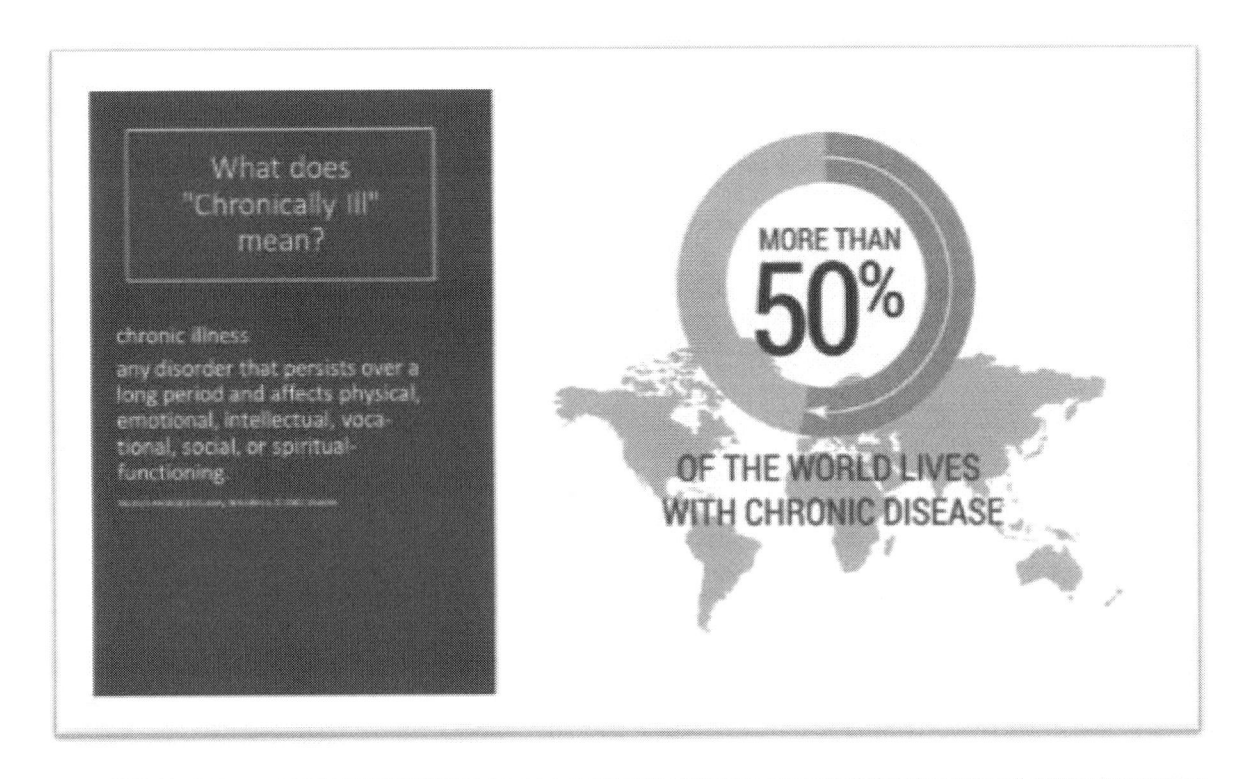

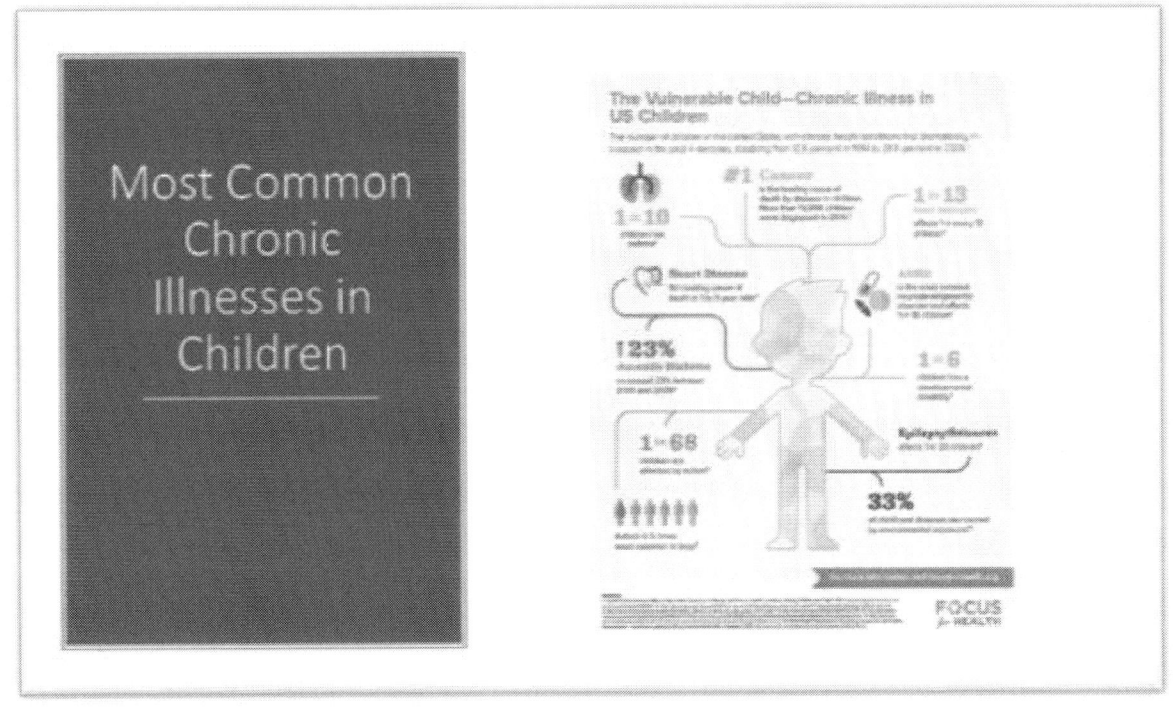

Asthma, Cystic fibrosis, Diabetes, Obesity, Malnutrition, Developmental disabilities, including attention-deficit/hyperactivity disorder (ADHD) and the autism spectrum disorders, Cerebral palsy, Consequences of low birth weight and prematurity, including chronic lung disease, retinopathy of prematurity (an eye disorder causing low vision or blindness), and developmental delays, Mental illnesses.

Most Common Chronic Illness at Mid-Life

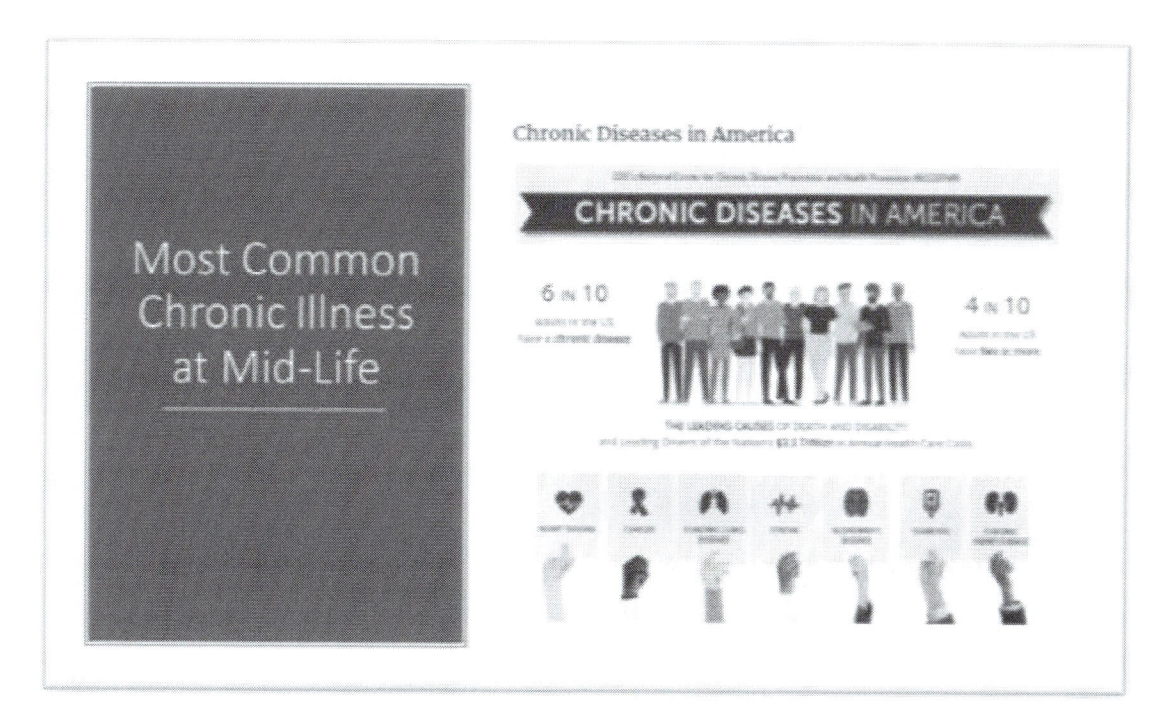

Chronic Diseases in America

6 in 10 adults in the U.S. have a chronic disease
4 in 10 adults in the U.S. have two or more

How common are chronic illnesses?

An estimated 57 million Americans had multiple chronic conditions in 2000, and that number is expected to reach 81 million by 2020—meaning that chronic illnesses have become the rule, not the exception. The most common chronic illnesses are: high blood pressure, high cholesterol, and rheumatological diseases.

Notes

_____

_____

_____

_____

_____

_____

Most Common Chronic Mental Illness – All Ages

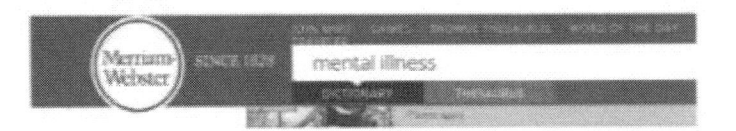

mental illness noun

variants: or **mental disorder** or less commonly **mental disease**

Definition of *mental illness*

: any of a broad range of medical conditions (such as major depression, schizophrenia, obsessive compulsive disorder, or panic disorder) that are marked primarily by sufficient disorganization of personality, mind, or emotions to impair normal psychological functioning and cause marked distress or disability and that are typically associated with a disruption in normal thinking, feeling, mood, behavior, interpersonal interactions, or daily functioning

- Depression
- Anxiety
- Eating Disorder
- A.D.D./A.D.H.D.
- Sexual Dysfunction*
- Substance Abuse*

Notes

_____

_____

_____

_____

_____

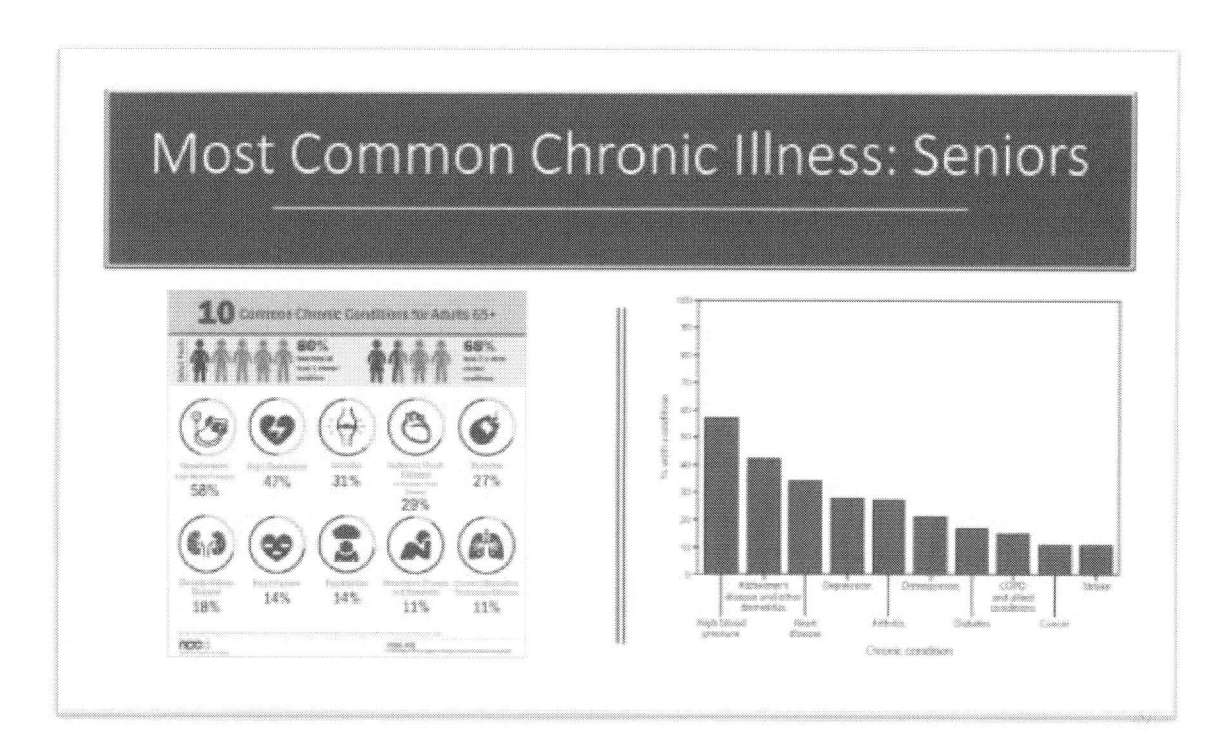

Most Common Chronic Illness: Seniors

High blood pressure (hypertension) affects 58% of seniors
High cholesterol affects 47% of seniors
Arthritis affects 31% of seniors
Coronary heart disease affects 29% of seniors
Diabetes affects 27% of senior
Chronic kidney disease (CKD) affects 18% of seniors
Heart failure affects 14% of seniors
Depression affects 14% of seniors
Alzheimer's disease and dementia affects 11% of seniors
Chronic obstructive pulmonary disease (COPD) affects 11% of seniors

Notes

_____

_____

_____

_____

_____

Titration with Whole Plant Products

Micro-dosing Strategies
- THC-sensitive individuals
- Supplement CBD regiments
- Short-term success

Common Patient Dosing
- One 10 mg nighttime dose
- 5 – 10 mg starting dose, 4 x day
- Continuous patient assessment of symptoms and side-effects
- Every 3 – 4 days, at least once per week, increase each daily dose by 5 – 10 mg
- Bulk up nighttime dose by doubling every 3 – 4 days

REPEAT ↑ ↗ ↓

CBD : THC
Goals? ... tions?

↑ CBD : THC ↓ | | ↓ CBD : THC ↑

- I don't want to feel high
- I need to stay clear-headed
- I wish for gentle mind, body, emotion relaxation

- I'm okay with some cognition changes
- I wish for moderate mind, body, emotion relaxation

- ...ay feeling high
- Side effects are acceptable
- I wish for deep mind, body, emotion relaxation

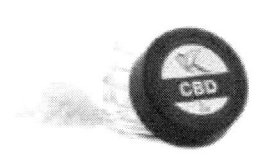

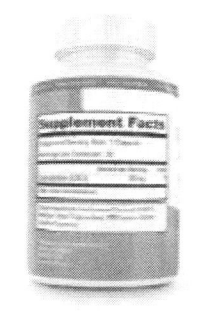

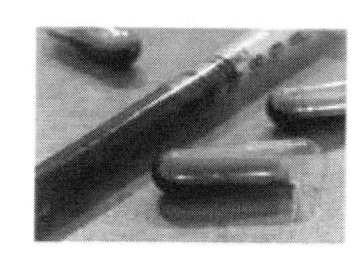

Whole Plant vs Isolates
Where's the *Entourage Effect*?

Scientific researchers note that cannabinoids can and should be isolated, so we can learn more about the individual functions of each. Certainly, some incredible pharmaceutical treatments await discovery with this approach and we do certainly learn more about each individual cannabinoid; but, it's also vital to understand that the scientists most educated on cannabinoids of any sort, researchers like Dr. Raphael Mechoulam, who discovered THC and the eCS, adamantly believe that the synergistic effects or *entourage effect* between cannabinoids and other cannabis compounds (like terpenes) is more effective than any one isolated cannabinoid; it is the combination of cannabinoids (THC, CBD, CBG, CBC, and others) that create specific health effects.

Notes

_____

_____

_____

_____

_____

_____

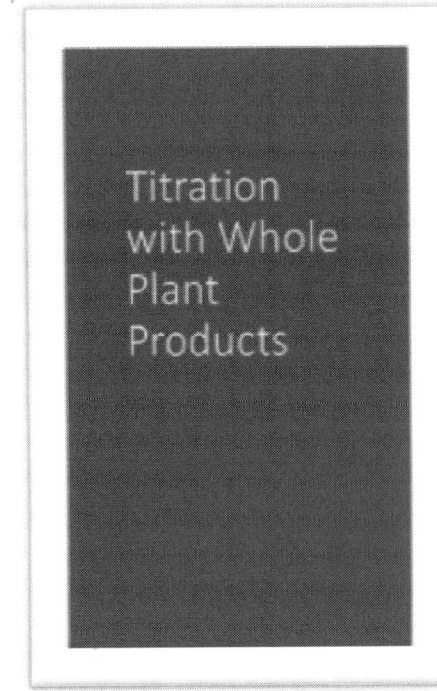

Titration with Whole Plant Products

Micro-dosing Strategies
- THC-sensitive individuals
- Supplement CBD regiments
- Short-term success

Common Patient Dosing
- One 10 mg nighttime dose
- 5 – 10 mg starting dose, 4 x day
- Continuous patient assessment of symptoms and side-effects
- Every 3 – 4 days, at least once per week, increase each daily dose by 5 – 10 mg
- Bulk up nighttime dose by doubling every 3 – 4 days

Currently there are two dosing theories in the cannabis world: micro-dosing strategies and common patient dosing.

Micro-Dosing
About 10 - 15% of the people who begin cannabis therapy and dedicatedly stick to the guidelines provided may still have an extreme sensitivity to cannabis therapy—maybe, not a full-blown adverse reaction, but they simply will not tolerate the THC or it's euphoric effects well. What do you do? You've come this far; will cannabis therapy work?

THC sensitive people (or the caregiver of one) need to know that even if the patient has THC-sensitivity, cannabis therapy may still be appropriate. In this case, micro-dosing may be a better option if the patient is using medical cannabis products. It will also help to try low THC options and avoid smoking cannabis.

Ideally, some one sensitive to THC should begin with a hemp oil extract product —and stay dedicated to help oil treatment for a period of several weeks. First, the patient may find CBD works effectively and they do not require more THC than hemp provides. At least, 20 – 30% of THC sensitive patients that try CBD hemp oil products may find success and have no need to secure actual medical cannabis products. Second, if the patient doesn't experience significant relief with the CBD product, they are still getting some cellular response. Give CBD a month or so, and if it's not ideal, then add 5 – 10 mgs doses of medical cannabis along with the CBD products. Also it is wise to add a choline supplement one or two days prior to starting medical cannabis (some THC) therapy. This will help reduce any euphoric side-effects including anxiety that often accompanies THC sensitivity.

Common Patient Dosing
For patients new to cannabis therapy, it is always wise to take the first dose at night—that way if the euphoric side-effects are too much the patient can sleep through the worst of it.

The first dose of cannabis should not exceed 10 mg—for most people, especially those not currently using cannabis, a 5 mg dose is best.

Ideally, the patient will take four (4) doses each day: morning, early afternoon, dinner time, and bed time. This allows cannabinoids to stay active in the patient's system, as well they will build up a storage of cannabinoids in their fat cells (the reason people fail drug tests).

In a perfect world, the patient will document their symptoms and side-effects so that others (Cannacians, caregivers, spouses, parents, etc) can help them understand how the cannabis is working.

Once per week—or as soon as every 3 -4 days—a patient can increase their individual daily doses by 5 – 10 mgs until they reach the 1 mg per kilo target. The patient should maintain this dose for a week or more before assessing how well cannabis therapy is working for them. A large percentage, perhaps as many as 80 – 90% of people, find sufficient relief at this initial target dose of 1 mg per kilo.

For patients who are trying to titrate up quickly (i.e., cancer patients), increasing the dose at night (much like beginning with a nighttime dose) will help determine if the side-effects will become 'too much' at the increased level.

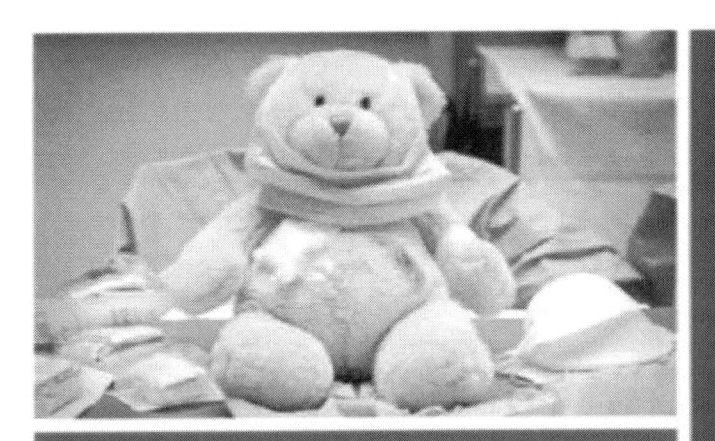

Dosing Strategies for Children

- Raw/Fresh
- THCa-based products except when 'rescue dosing' is necessary
- Broad-based Cannabinoid Profiles
- Sublingual for Rapid Relief, Edible for Long-Term Relief

Dosing Strategies for Adults & Seniors

- Sublingual, Vapor or Smoking for Rapid Relief
- Edible (minimum of One per Day) for Long-Term Relief
- Layer Cannabis Therapies
- Always include a Topical Cannabis Product in regiment
- Largest Doses of THC before bed
- Slow and Steady approaches are tolerated best

Objectives

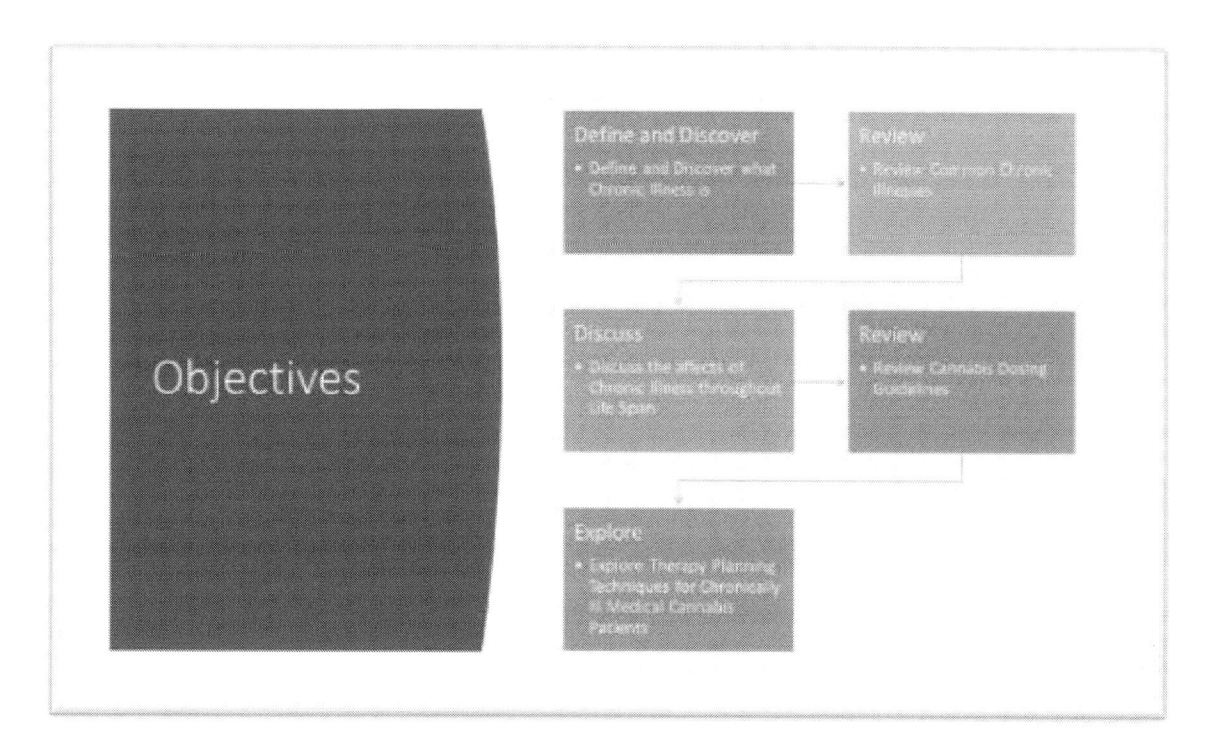

Define and Discover
- Define and Discover what Chronic Illness is

Review
- Review Common Chronic Illnesses

Discuss
- Discuss the affects of Chronic Illness throughout Life Span

Review
- Review Cannabis Dosing Guidelines

Explore
- Explore Therapy Planning Techniques for Chronically Ill Medical Cannabis Patients

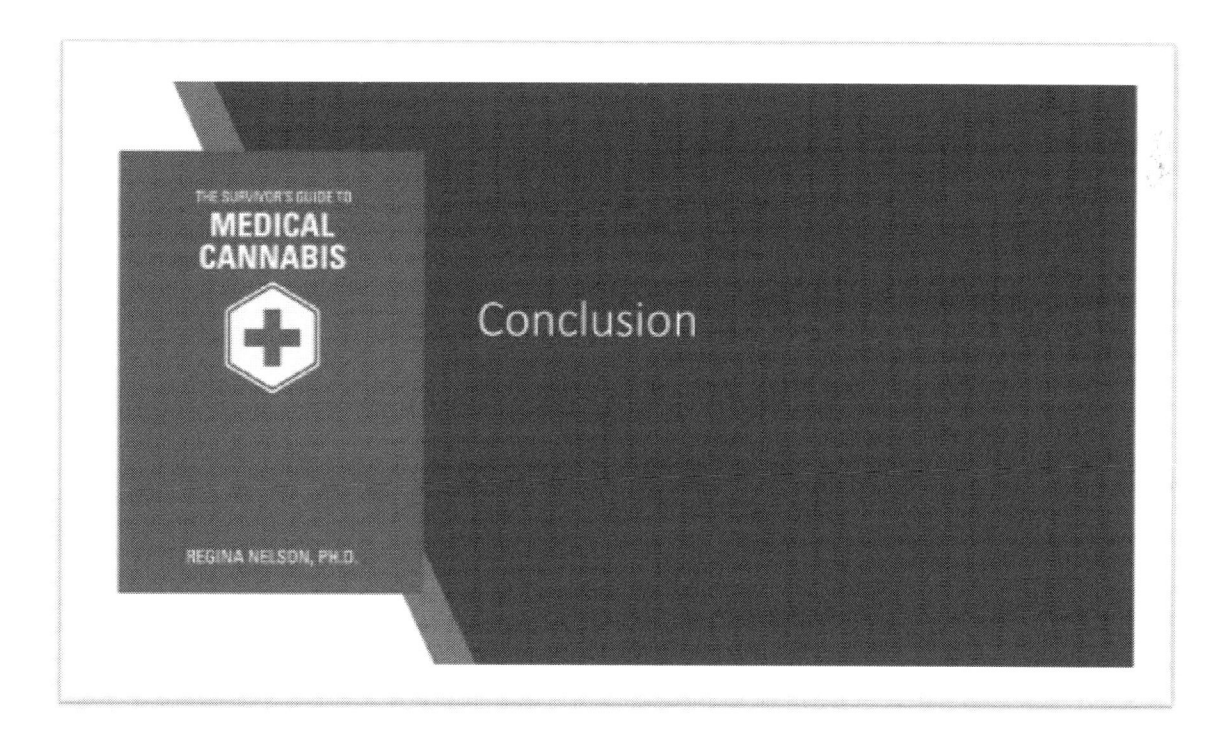

THE SURVIVOR'S GUIDE TO
MEDICAL CANNABIS

REGINA NELSON, PH.D.

Conclusion

Notes

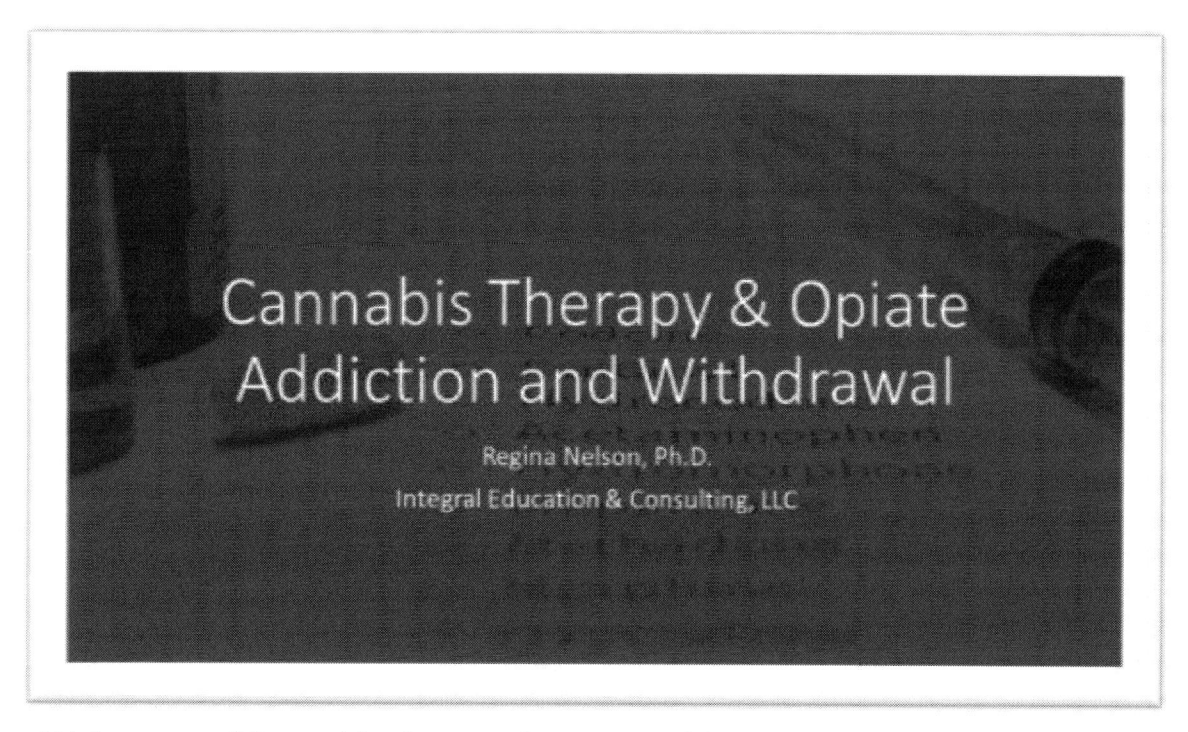

Cannabis Therapy & Opiate Addiction and Withdrawal

Regina Nelson, Ph.D.
Integral Education & Consulting, LLC

Welcome to "Cannabis Therapy & Opiate Addication and Withdrawal." This is the third module of the Cannacian™ Level Three Certification program.

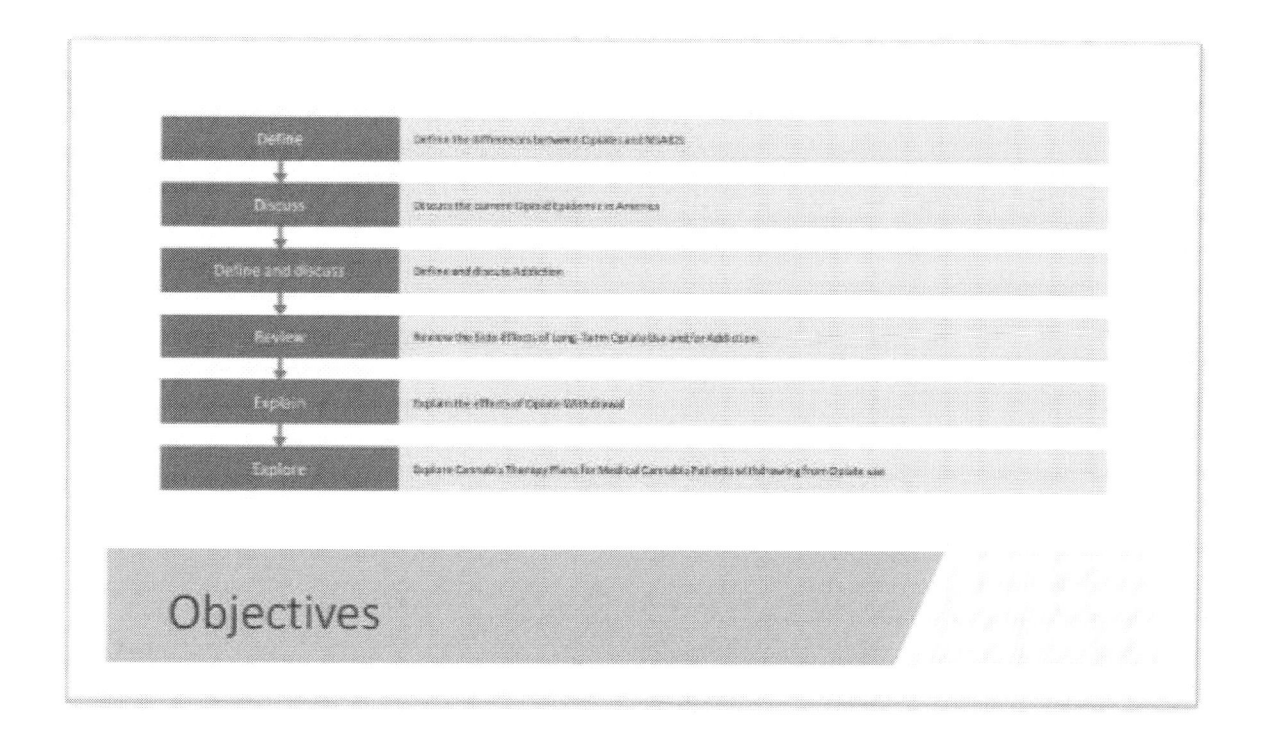

Objectives

- **Define** — Define the differences between Opiates and NSAIDS
- **Discuss** — Discuss the current Opioid Epidemic in America
- **Define and discuss** — Define and discuss Addiction
- **Review** — Review the Side Effects of Long-Term Opiate Use and/or Addiction
- **Explain** — Explain the effects of Opiate Withdrawal
- **Explore** — Explore Cannabis Therapy Plans for Medical Cannabis Patients withdrawing from Opiate use

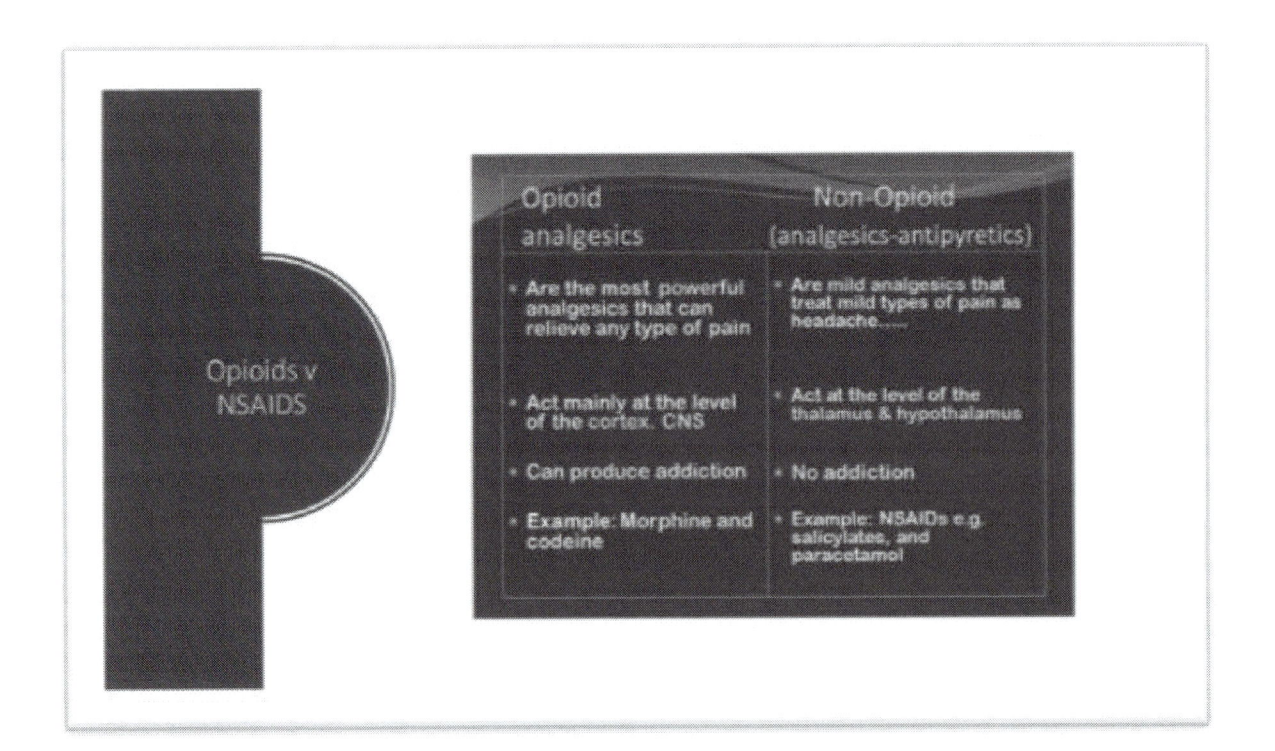

Opioid analgesics	Non-Opioid (analgesics-antipyretics)
Are the most powerful analgesics that can relieve any type of pain	Are mild analgesics that treat mild types of pain as headache......
Act mainly at the level of the cortex, CNS	Act at the level of the thalamus & hypothalamus
Can produce addiction	No addiction
Example: Morphine and codeine	Example: NSAIDs e.g. salicylates, and paracetamol

Opioids v NSAIDS

OPIOIDS VS. NSAIDS

There are two main categories of pain medications, opioids and non-steroidal anti-inflammatory drugs (NSAIDs). Although these two categories of drugs work differently, they do share one thing in common: both are derivatives of natural products. NSAID commonly known as Aspirin was developed by **Bayer** (Leverkusen, Germany). It is a synthetic version of an extract from willow tree bark. Opioids are synthetic versions of opium and morphine, which come from poppy flowers.

It takes a couple of weeks to become physically dependent on an opioid, but that varies by individual. If you take an opioid for a day or two, it should not be a problem and, generally, you will not become addicted. However, some studies show even the first dose of an opioid can have physiological effects.

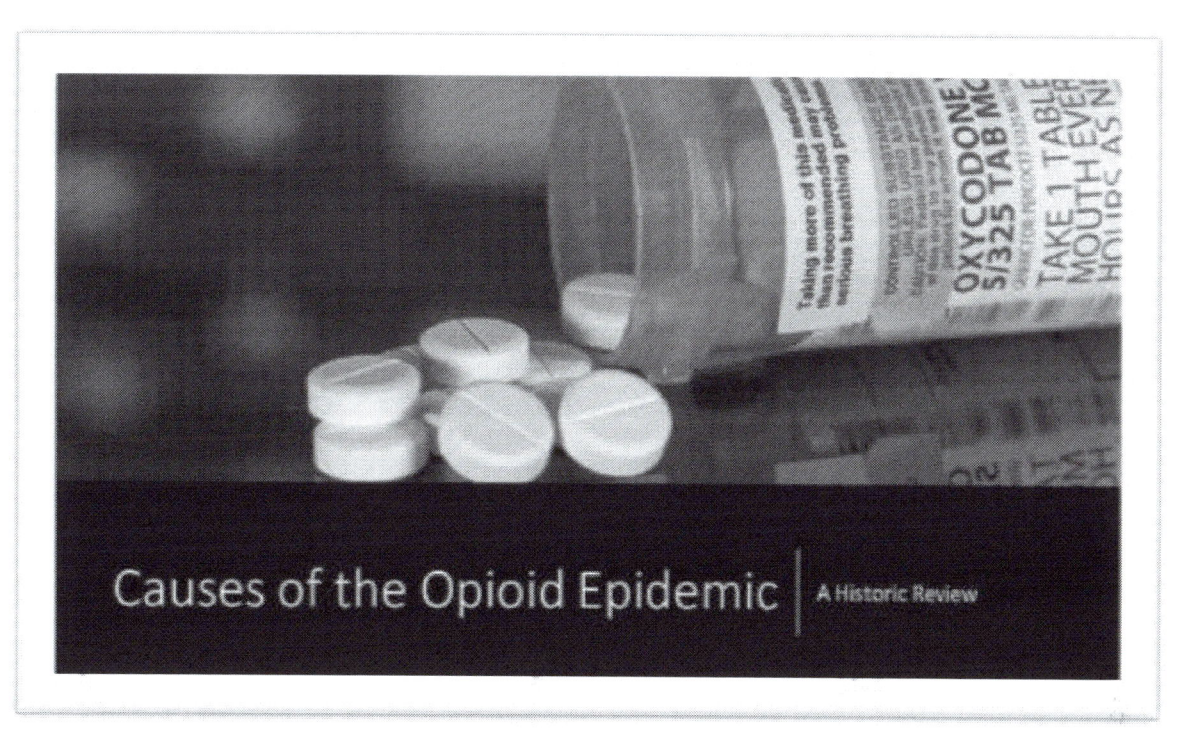

Causes of the Opioid Epidemic | A Historic Review

Deaths caused by drug overdose have been continually increasing over the past several decades, roughly two-thirds of these due to opioid use equating to more than 91 people a day, dead from an opioid overdose—
that's truly terrifying.

The majority of people addicted to opiates did not begin them with a illicit drugs, such as heroin or cocaine. Rather, most begin their addiction to opioids in the form of prescriptive opioids legally prescribed by their own doctor for pain.

Synthetic and semi-synthetic opioids include methadone, oxycodone, hydrocodone, hydromorphone, and oxymorphone. Examples of legal natural opioids are morphine and codeine.

U.S. Statistics (2016)

- 116 people died from opioid-related overdoses each day.
- Over 42,000 people died from opioid overdoses over the course of the year.
- 1 million people had an opioid disorder.
- 17,087 deaths were caused by overdoses on commonly prescribed opioids.
- 19,413 deaths resulted from use of other synthetic opioids other than methadone.
- 15,469 deaths were attributed to heroin overdose

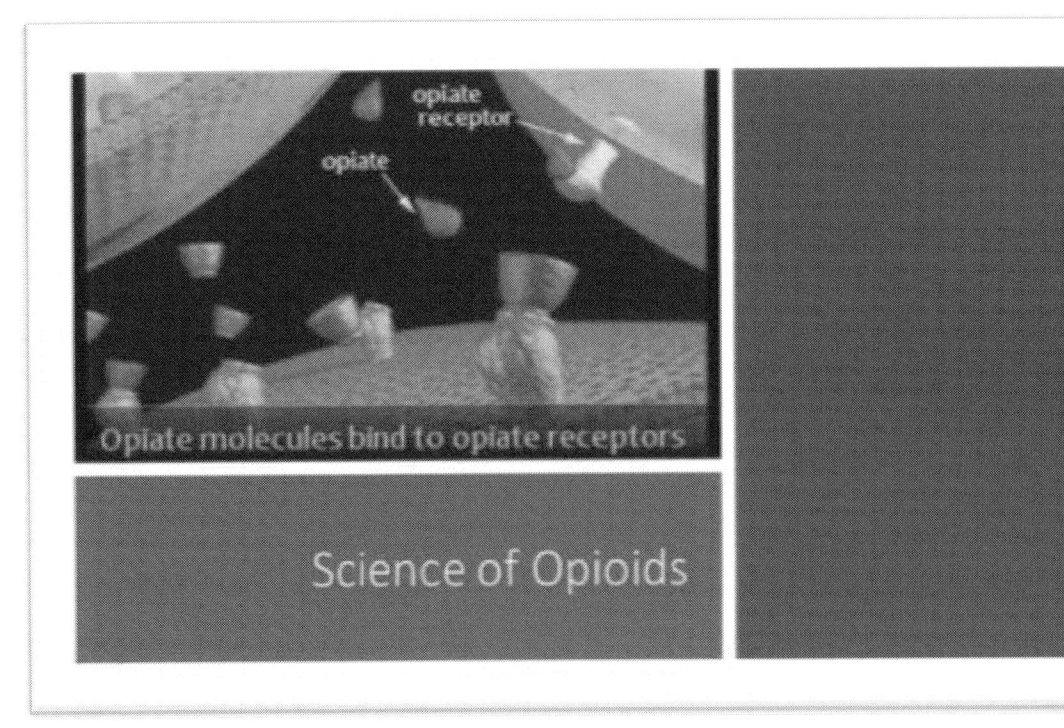

Opiate molecules bind to opiate receptors

Science of Opioids

Prescription opioid drugs (such as oxycodone and hydrocodone) and heroin work through the same mechanism of action. Opioids reduce the perception of pain by binding to opioid receptors, which are found on cells in the brain and in other organs in the body. The binding of these drugs to opioid receptors in reward regions in the brain produces a sense of well-being, while stimulation of opioid receptors in deeper brain regions results in drowsiness and respiratory depression, which can lead to overdose deaths.

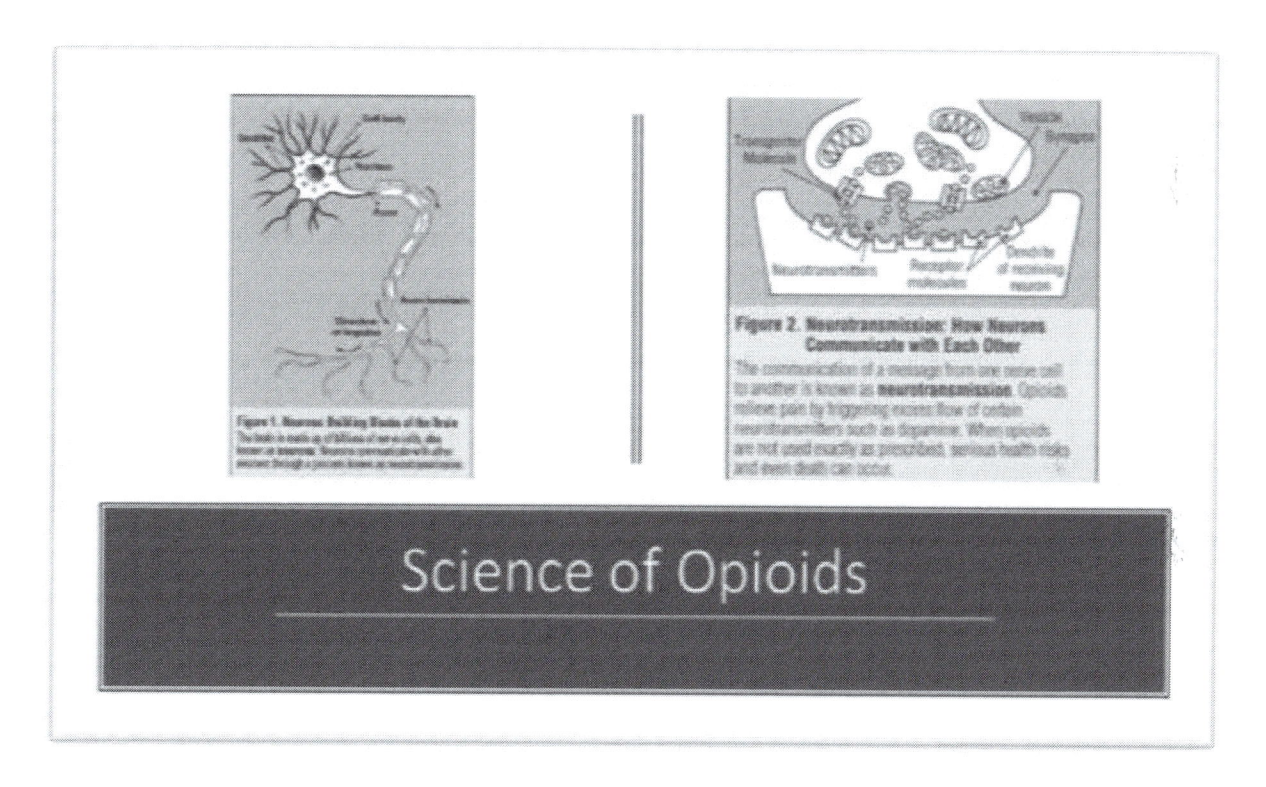

Science of Opioids

Opioids work by attaching to specific proteins called opioid *receptors* that are found in the brain, spinal cord, and gastrointestinal tract. Opioids relieve pain by triggering excess flow of certain neurotransmitters such as *dopamine*. Yet, when opioids are over used or abused serious health risks, including overdose and death, can occur.

Defining Addiction

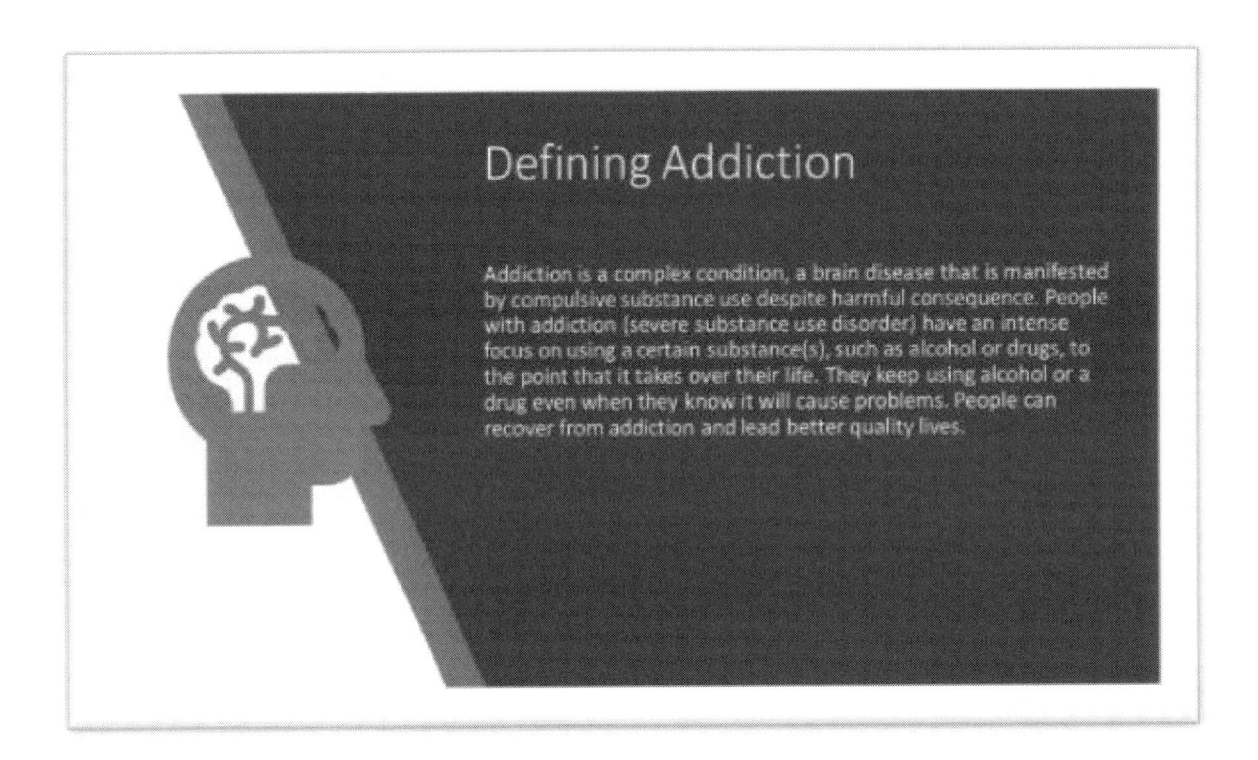

Addiction is a complex condition, a brain disease that is manifested by compulsive substance use despite harmful consequence. People with addiction (severe substance use disorder) have an intense focus on using a certain substance(s), such as alcohol or drugs, to the point that it takes over their life. They keep using alcohol or a drug even when they know it will cause problems. People can recover from addiction and lead better quality lives.

When we talk about addiction or opioid use disorder, often people refer to a syndrome of symptoms. The syndrome has features, such as the person using the opioid is giving up other things in their life, and the use of the drug starts to impact them (their health, their relationships). They crave the drug, and the use of it starts to impact their whole life. Their life becomes organized around the use of opioids.

In addition, with opioids (and other drugs as well, such as alcohol) there is something else — physical dependence, a physiological adaptation that occurs when using a substance. When the person stops taking the drug, they experience withdrawal. Consider caffeine, for example — if you stop consuming it, you can develop a withdrawal headache and flulike symptoms. It is important to understand that you can be physically dependent on a substance but you don't necessarily have problematic use. A cancer patient with chronic pain may be physically dependent but not addicted.

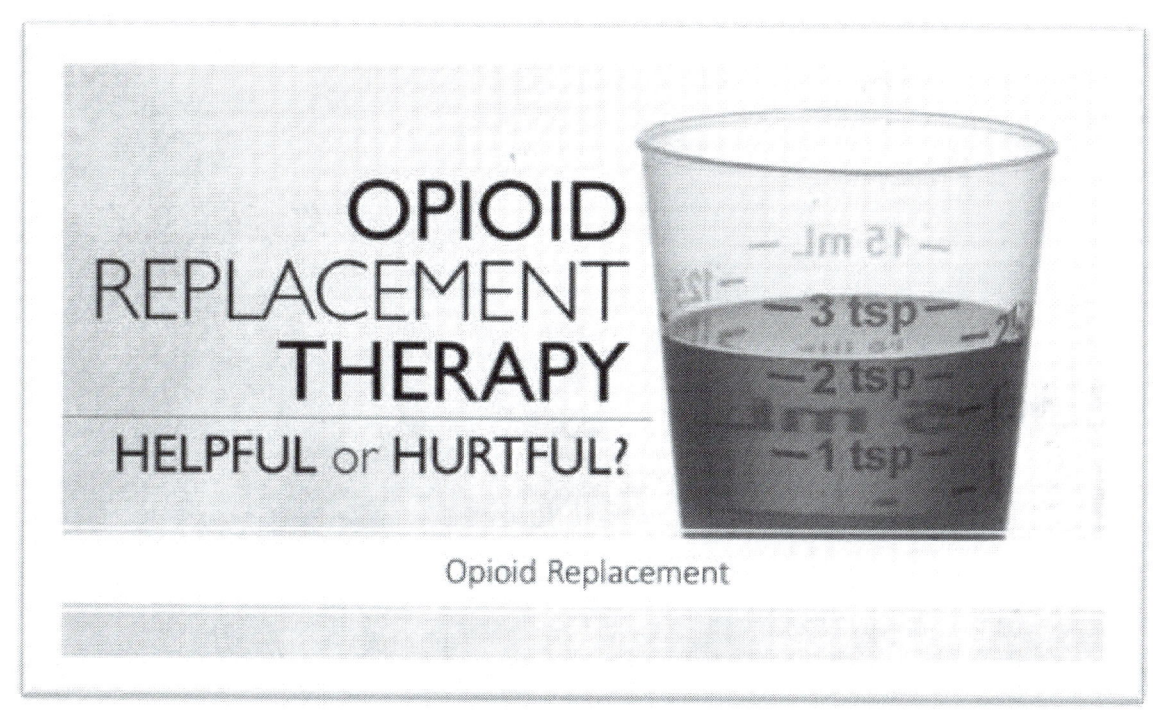

OPIOID REPLACEMENT THERAPY
HELPFUL or HURTFUL?

Opioid Replacement

Methadone, a long-acting narcotic painkiller, fits into the same brain receptors as opioids but doesn't produce the euphoric "high" the opioid drugs do. It also can block opioids from attaching to the receptors, if a person relapses and takes an opioid after having taken methadone.

Naltrexone, approved to treat opioid addiction in 1984 and alcohol addiction in 1994, binds to the receptors and blocks them altogether so that opioids can't attach. Because naltrexone doesn't activate the receptors at all, though, it won't prevent withdrawal symptoms, and patient compliance with taking it regularly has historically been low. In recent years, naltrexone has been available in an injection — Vivitrol — that's taken once a month.

Buprenorphine — sometimes combined with naloxone in Suboxone — fits into the opioid receptors, but it's not a perfect fit, so the receptor only partially "fires." The body is tricked into thinking it has opioids, but buprenorphine won't produce a euphoric high or depress the respiratory system.

Symptoms of Opioid Withdrawal

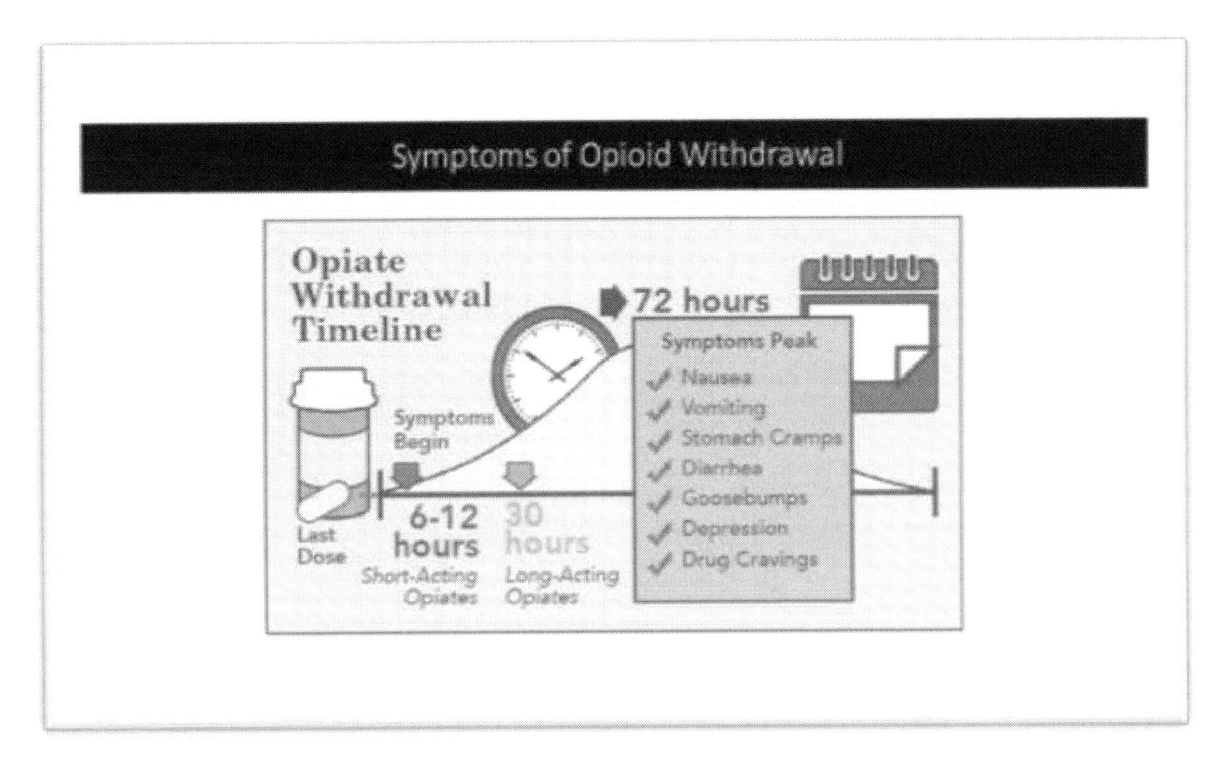

Opiate Withdrawal Timeline

Last Dose → Symptoms Begin: 6-12 hours (Short-Acting Opiates), 30 hours (Long-Acting Opiates)

72 hours — Symptoms Peak:
- Nausea
- Vomiting
- Stomach Cramps
- Diarrhea
- Goosebumps
- Depression
- Drug Cravings

Prolonged use of opioids changes the way nerve receptors work in the brain, which eventually become dependent on the drug to function. When an opioid user stops or decreases opioid use, it can lead to physical symptoms of withdrawal which can range from mild to moderate or severe.

These symptoms may include:
- Muscle aches
- Restlessness
- Anxiety
- Eyes that tear up
- Runny nose
- Excessive sweating
- Inability to sleep
- Yawning very often
- Diarrhea
- Abdominal cramping
- Goose bumps on the skin
- Nausea and vomiting
- Dilated pupils and possibly blurry vision
- Rapid heartbeat
- High blood pressure

Opioid withdrawal symptoms can be very uncomfortable, and opioid users may continue to take their drugs to avoid the physical withdrawal effects.

Long-Term Effects of Opioids

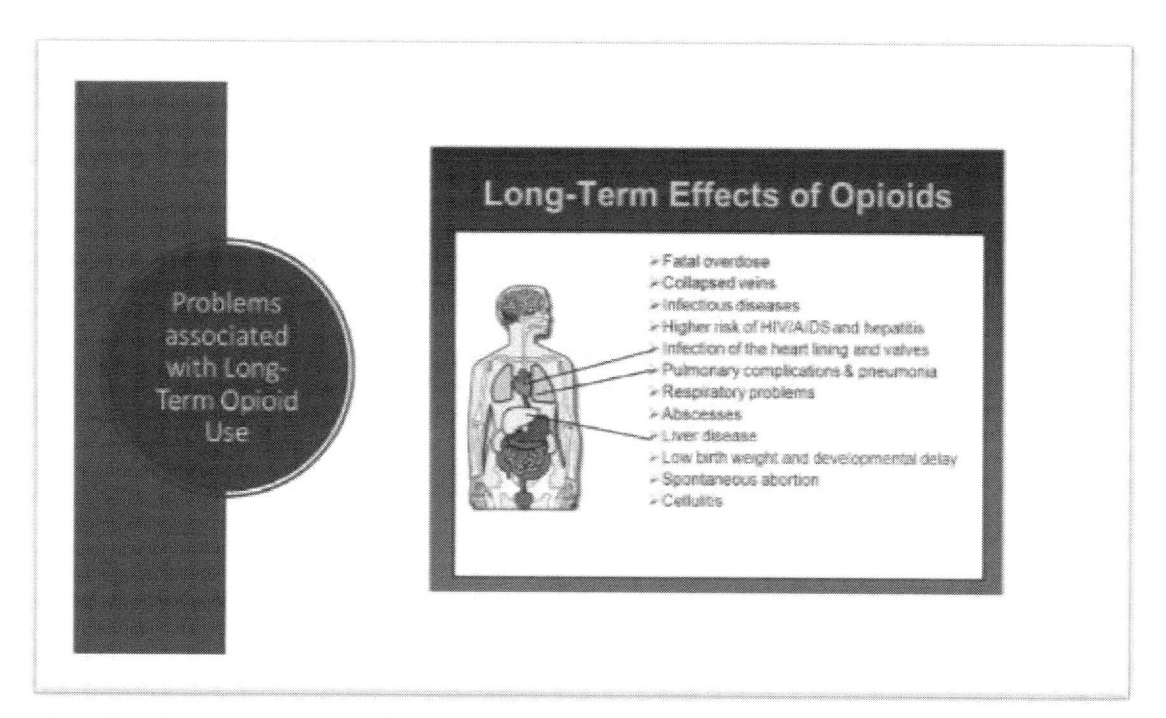

Problems associated with Long-Term Opioid Use

- Fatal overdose
- Collapsed veins
- Infectious diseases
- Higher risk of HIV/AIDS and hepatitis
- Infection of the heart lining and valves
- Pulmonary complications & pneumonia
- Respiratory problems
- Abscesses
- Liver disease
- Low birth weight and developmental delay
- Spontaneous abortion
- Cellulitis

Studies have suggested opioid abuse can not only lower the level of the chemical used to transmit opioid signals, but it can also damage the particular circuit that carries the signals from the prefrontal cortex to the reward center. This can disconnect the part of the brain responsible for insight and judgment—the prefrontal cortex—and the "reward center" (I.e. mesolimbic system) that trigger dopamine causing the inability to use judgement to restrain bad impulses. The good news is that these connections can reform, but that takes time—about 2 years for most people.

The most common side effects of opioid use are constipation and nausea. Other common side effects of opioid use include sedation, dizziness, vomiting, tolerance, physical dependence, and respiratory depression.

Drug Cravings

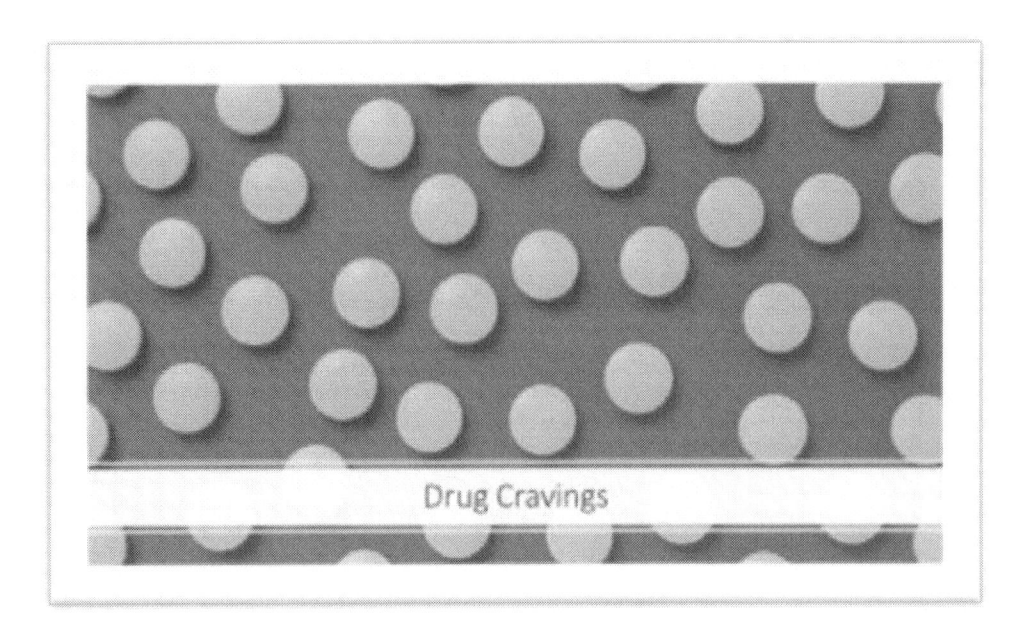

Cravings are powerful psychological and physiological reactions in the brain that create strong memories of drug use in an addict that can last for years —simply, an intense desire for the opioid.

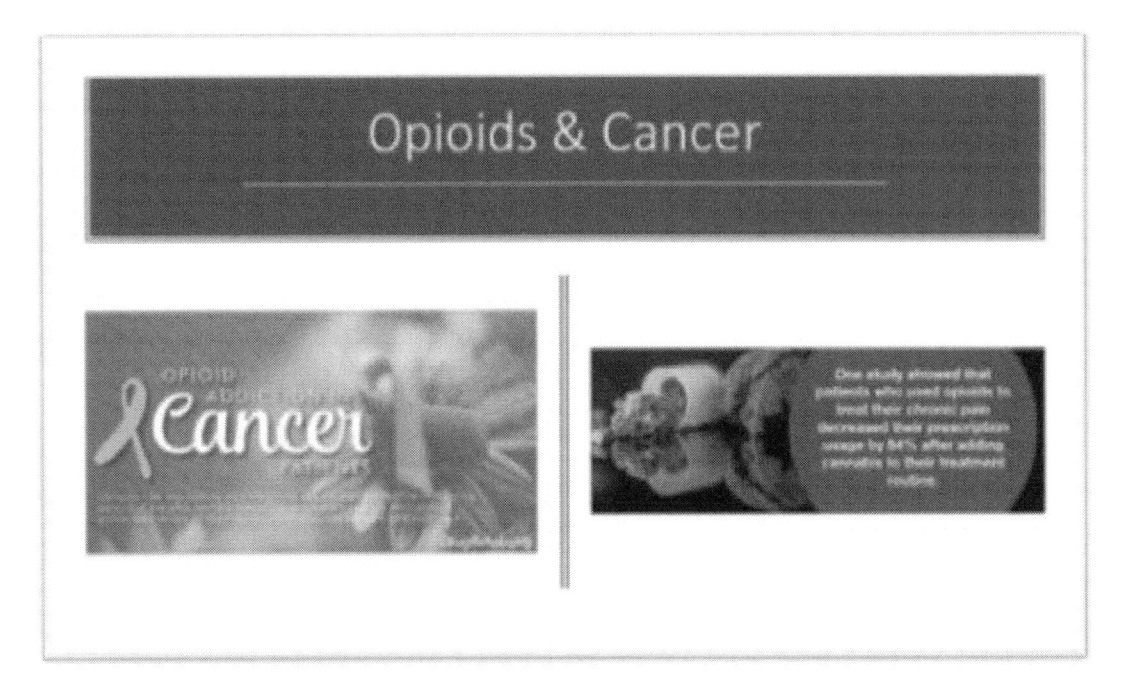

Opioids & Cancer

Recent studies show that lung cancer cells with additional opioid receptors grow more than twice as fast as tumor cells without extra receptors when transplanted into mice. These lung cancer cells are also 20 times more likely to spread to other sites within the body.

Overdose: Opioid v Cannabis

In 2014, almost 2 million people in the U.S. were abusing or were addicted to opioid drugs. More than 21,000 died from overdoses in the same year.

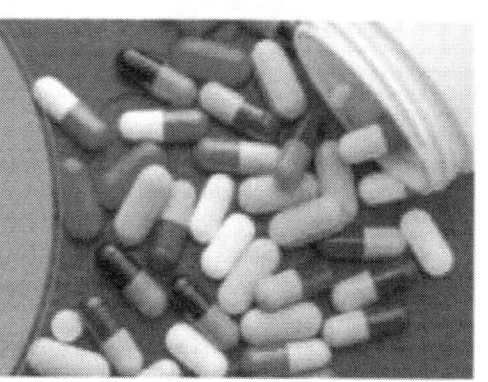

Science of Cannabis

- Every Human has an Endocannabinoid System

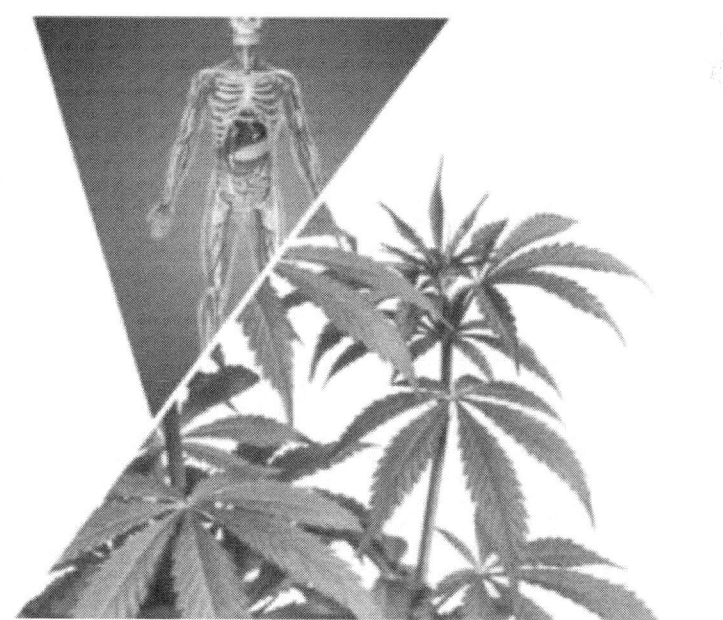

Cannabis Therapy & Opioid Withdrawal

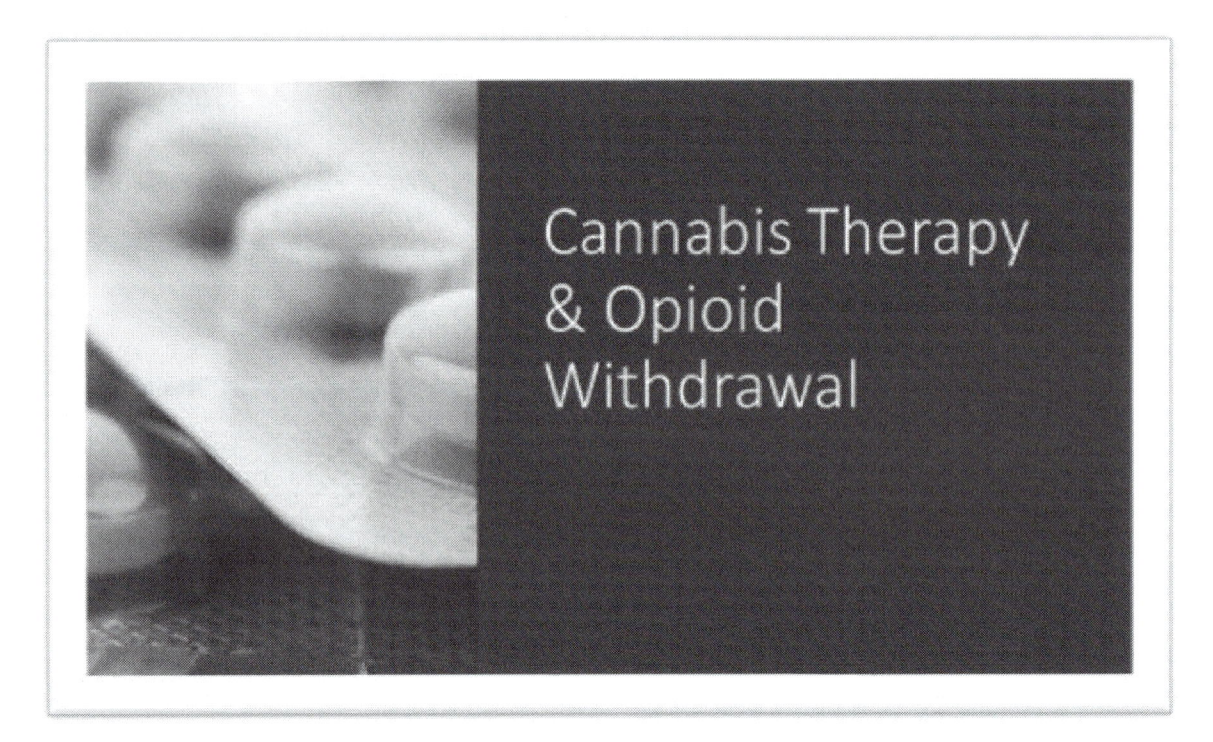

- 1 – 10 mg per kilo
  - Both THC or CBD rich therapies may be helpful for opioid withdrawal and pain control
  - Initial Target Dose is 1 mg per kilo
  - 5 mg per kilo common withdrawal dose
    - Vapor for acute relief
    - Edible/Capsule base dose
    - Topicals for acute & long-term relief
-

Notes

Chronic Pain

- 1 – 10 mg per kilo
  - Both THC or CBD rich therapies may be helpful for opioid withdrawal and pain control
  - Initial Target Dose is 1 mg per kilo
  - 5 mg per kilo common withdrawal dose
    - Vapor for acute relief
    - Edible/Capsule base dose
    - Topicals for acute & long-term relief

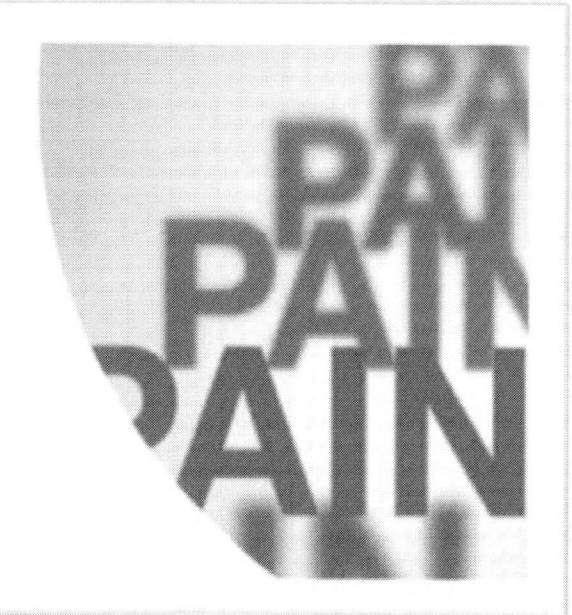

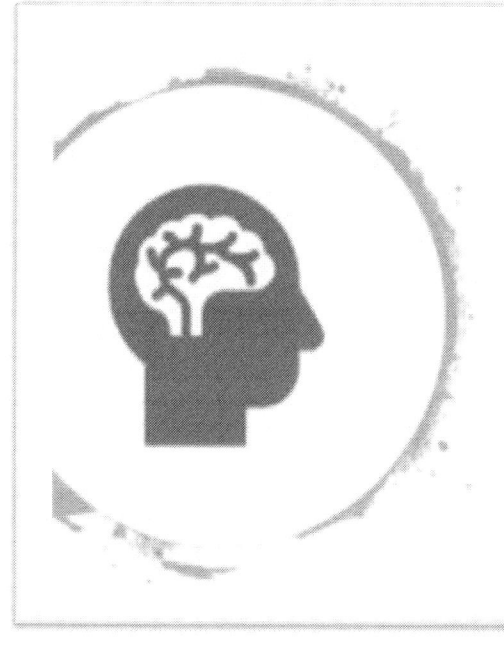

Objectives Revisited

- Define the differences between Opiates and NSAIDS
- Discuss the current Opioid Epidemic in America
- Define and discuss Addiction
- Review the Side-Effects of Long-Term Opiate Use and/or Addiction
- Explain the effects of Opiate Withdrawal
- Explore Cannabis Therapy Plans for Medical Cannabis Patients withdrawing from Opiate use

Notes

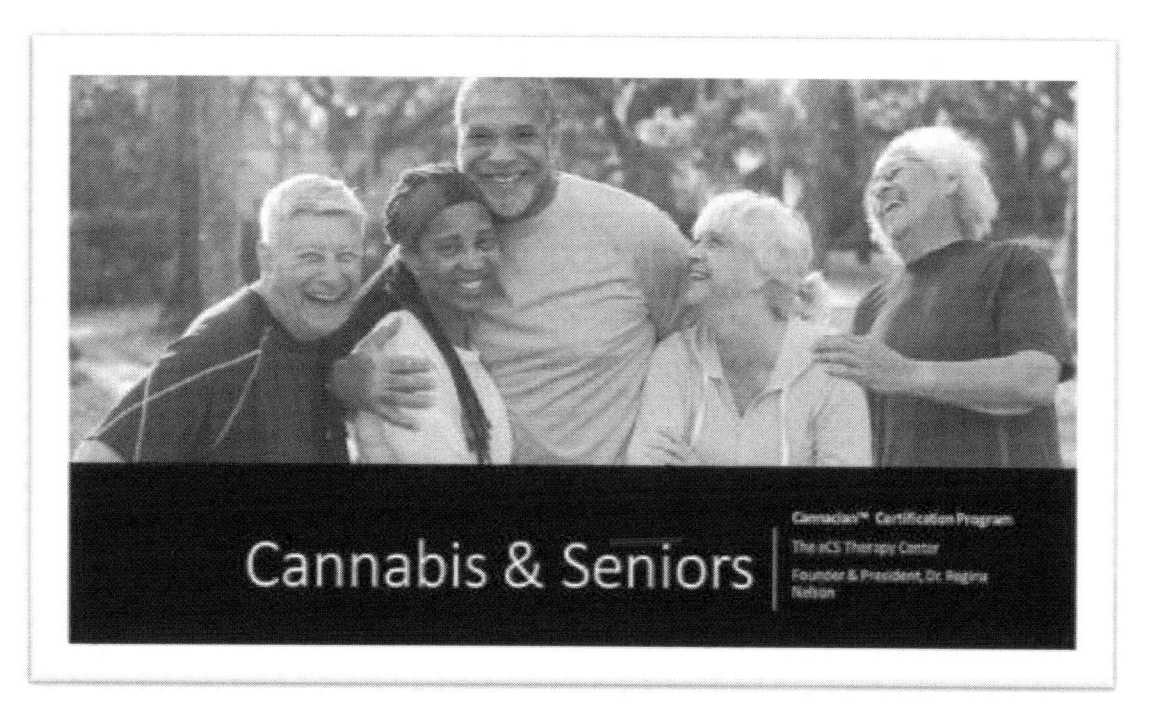

Cannabis & Seniors

Cannacian™ Certification Program
The aCS Therapy Center
Founder & President, Dr. Regina Nelson

Welcome to "Cannabis & Seniors" the fourth and final module of the Cannacian™ Level Three Certification program. It is also the final module in the Cannacian™ Certification program. Congratulations! You've nearly completed the program!

Seniors are the fastest growing population of medical cannabis patients. This means it is an important population to focus on educating and supporting as a Cannacian™.

Objectives

- Define "Senior" and discuss the largest growing population of cannabis patients
- Review common health challenges for seniors
- Discuss developing cannabis therapy plans for senior patients
- Address healthy seniors and cannabis

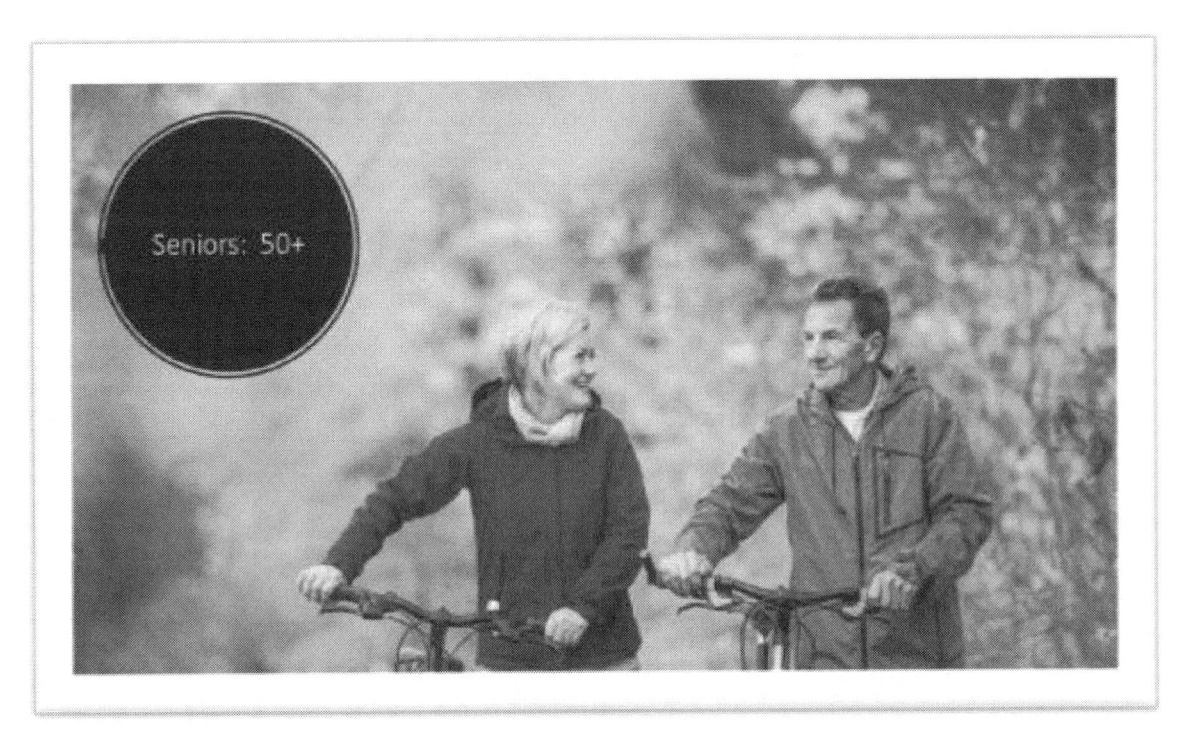

Typically the senior population is defined as adults aged 65 or older. But like many restaurant menus we are going to allow seniors to be 50+ because the onset of many of the most common senior health issues begin occurring in the 50's.

In 2014, 14.5% (46.3 million) of the US population was aged 65 or older and the senior population is projected to reach 23.5% (98 million) by 2060.

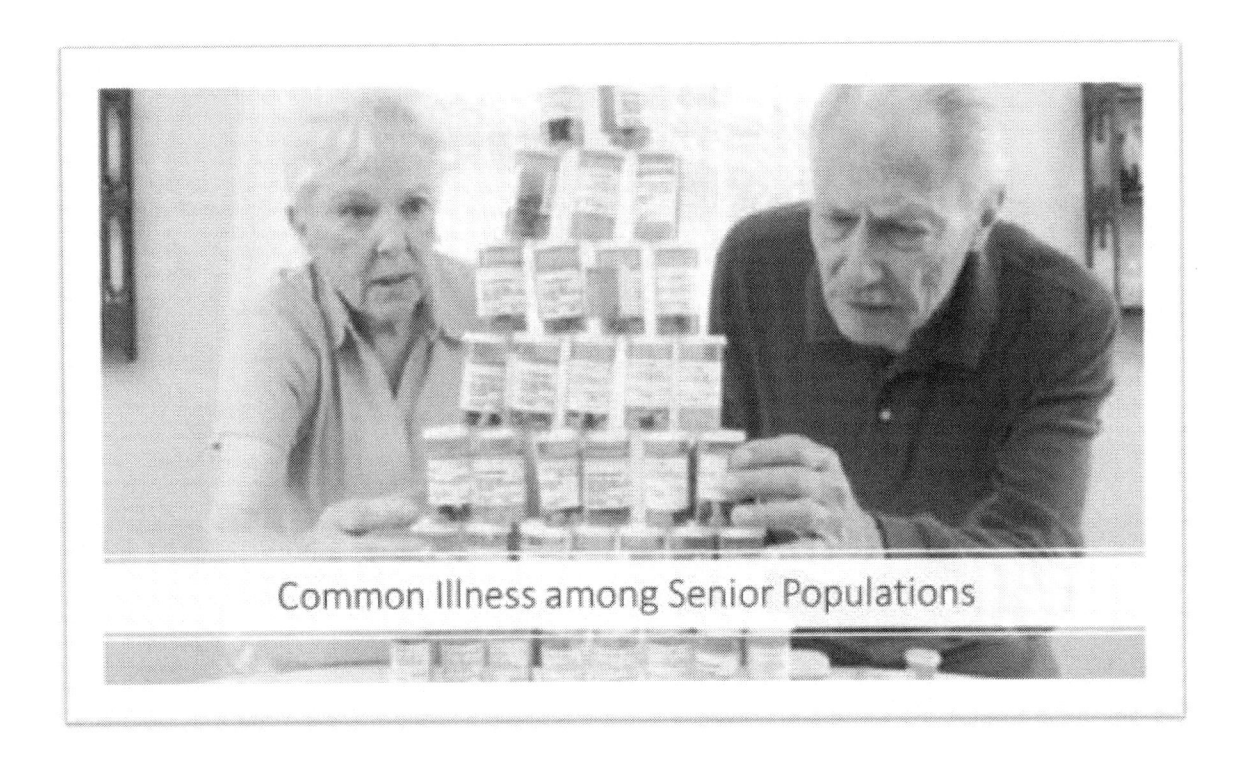

Arthritis is the #1 health concern among seniors 65+

Heart disease: so being able to eat right and exercise is vital to senior health

Cancer is the 2nd leading cause of death among seniors

Chronic respiratory distress affects more than 10% of both senior men and women

More than 10% of seniors are affected by Alzheimer's disease, and a larger population by other dementia related issues

By 2020 it is expected that osteopososis will affect 64 Million Americans, most seniors

More than ¼ of the senior population lives with diabetes

Injuries from accidental falls are common among seniors

Obesity, Depression, and poor oral health are also common among seniors.

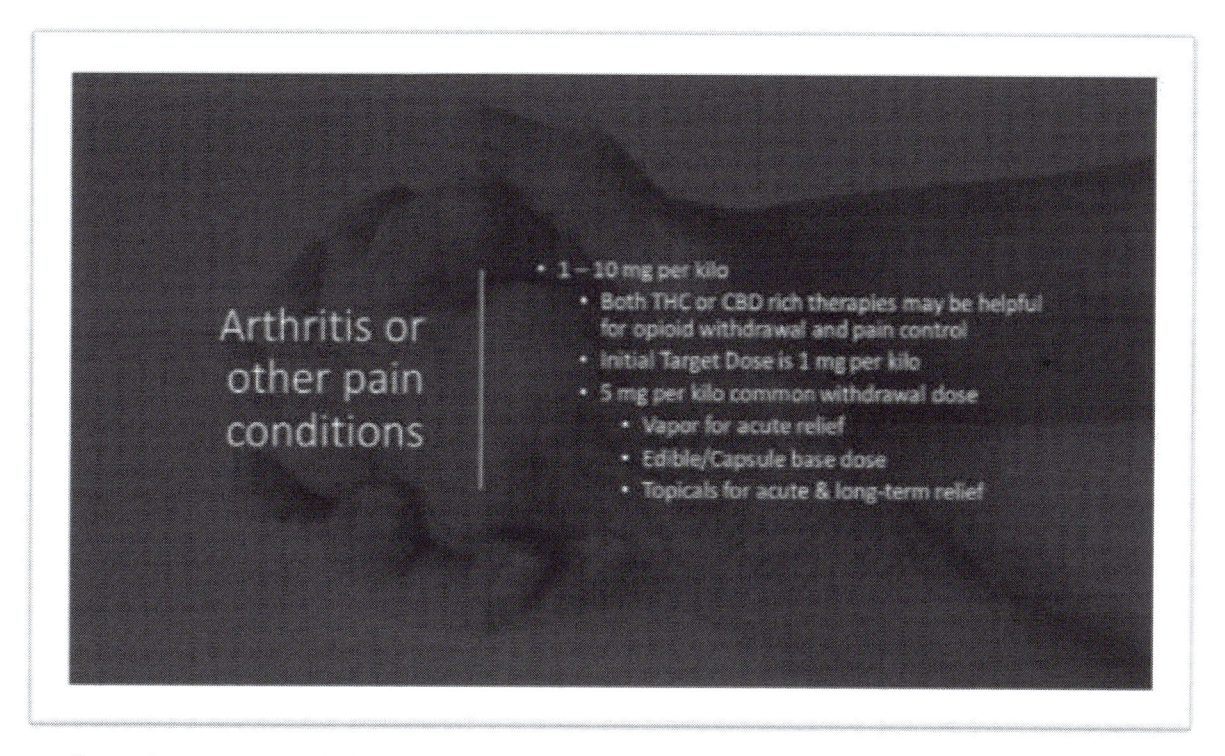

Arthritis or other pain conditions

- 1 – 10 mg per kilo
- Both THC or CBD rich therapies may be helpful for opioid withdrawal and pain control
- Initial Target Dose is 1 mg per kilo
- 5 mg per kilo common withdrawal dose
  - Vapor for acute relief
  - Edible/Capsule base dose
  - Topicals for acute & long-term relief

Follow the pain guidelines we disuccsed in the Opiate Addiction & Withdrawal module. Assure that cannabinoid spectrums are broad and if possible use THC in THCa form. Cautiously titrate the patient as a caregiver observes how they adjust to regular daily dosing. Instead of edibles as a primary source of cannabinoids, a tincture or suspension will be easier for patients and caregivers to gauge.

For patients with chronic pain issues it is suggested that they layer cannabis therapies—meaning they should use cannabis in a variety of different ways for maximum relief. For example, a consistent dose of indica-dominant cannabis oil in the 1-5 mg per kilo range each day may reduce pain symptoms considerably regardless of the condition or injury contributing to the pain. The addition of topical products on a regular basis, and smoking/vaporizing cannabis when symptoms are most acute (i.e., patient has a flare), will also provide a great deal of relief. For those new to cannabis therapy, beginning with a combination of tincture/ suspension or an edible at a very low dose taken several times a day, a topical salve applied several times per day, and vaporizing if the pain is acute will provide the best relief. For those with major pain issues, the range of 5-10 mgs of cannabis oil per kilo per day may be required for symptoms to be managed effectively.

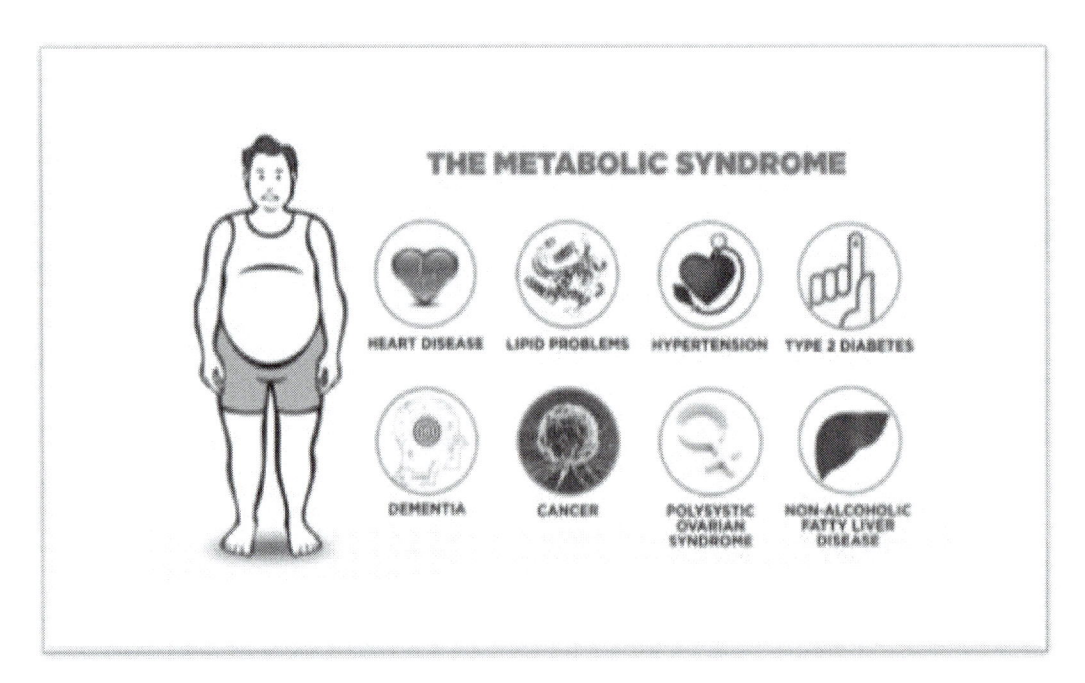

THE METABOLIC SYNDROME

HEART DISEASE · LIPID PROBLEMS · HYPERTENSION · TYPE 2 DIABETES

DEMENTIA · CANCER · POLYCYSTIC OVARIAN SYNDROME · NON-ALCOHOLIC FATTY LIVER DISEASE

Metabolism is the process your body uses to get or make energy from the food you eat. Food is made up of proteins, carbohydrates, and fats. Chemicals in your digestive system break the food parts down into sugars and acids, your body's fuel. Your body can use this fuel right away, or it can store the energy in your body tissues, such as your liver, muscles, and body fat.

Your metabolic system is actually a series of systems working as a team. They include your pancreas, liver, thyroid, and hypothalamus. Each part plays a very specific role such as turning food into energy, processing that energy, and digesting food.

[handwritten note: HORMONE REGULATION]

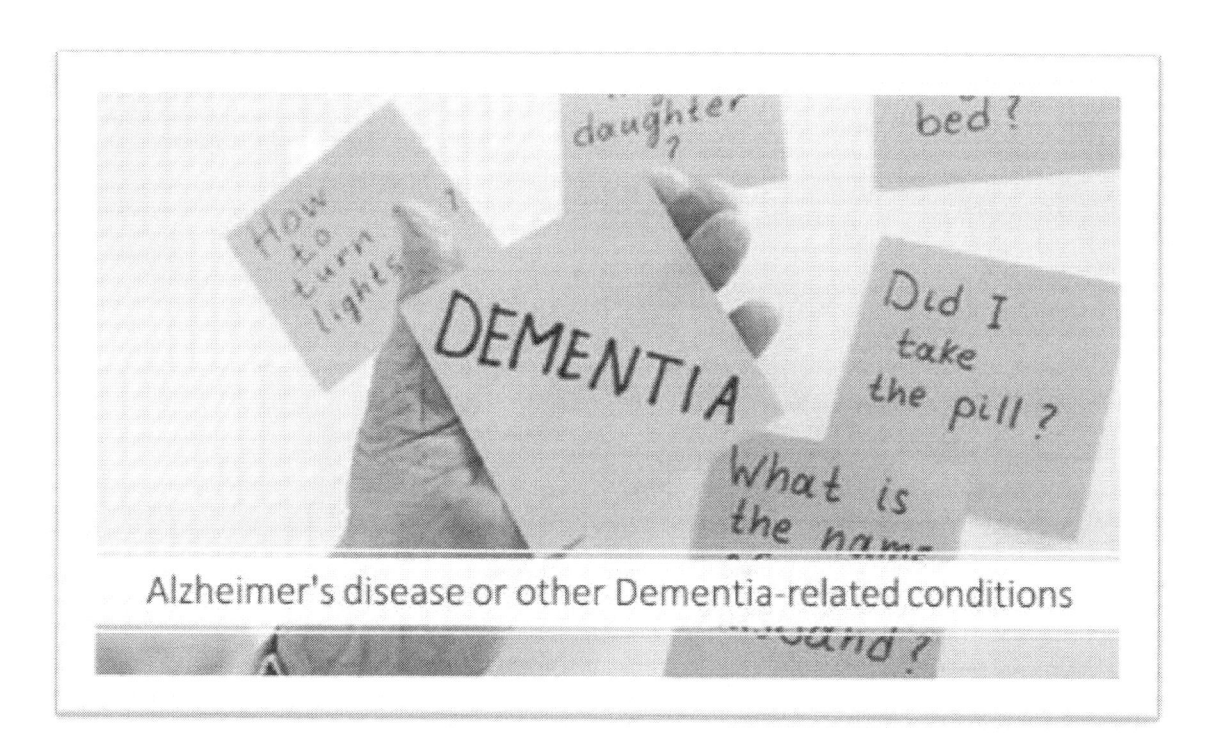

Alzheimer's disease or other Dementia-related conditions

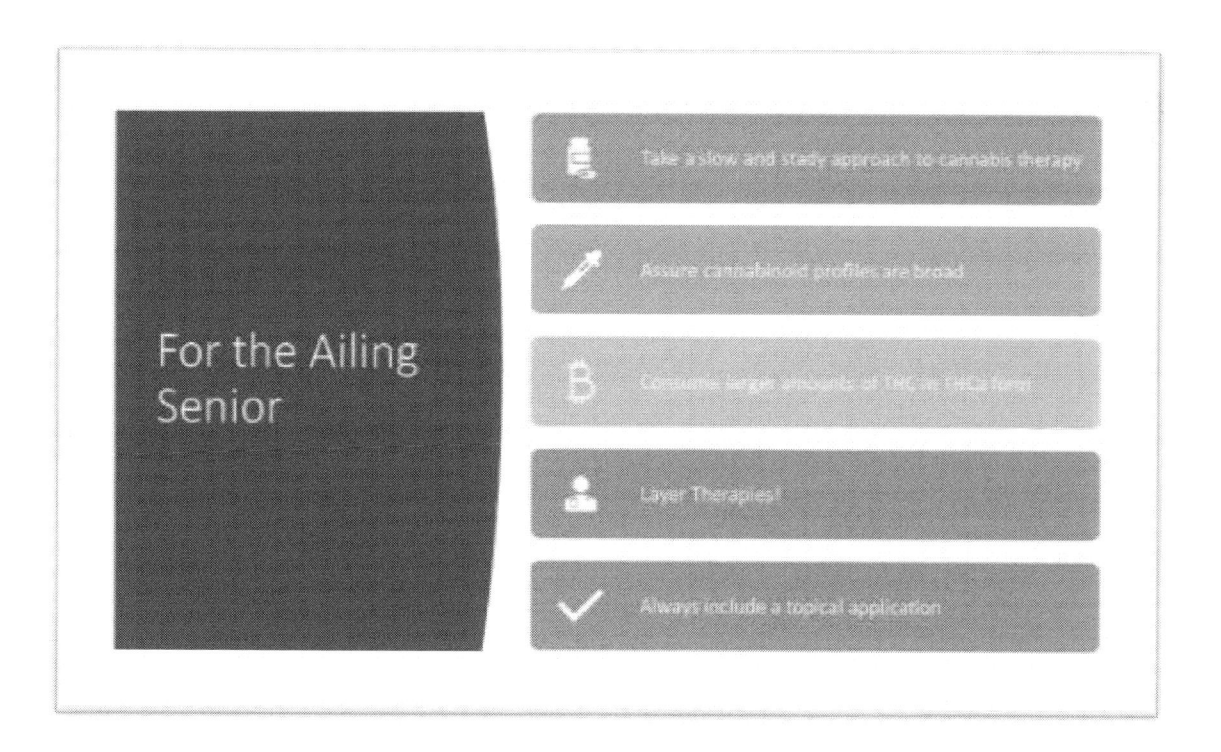

For the Ailing Senior

- Take a slow and steady approach to cannabis therapy
- Assure cannabinoid profiles are broad
- Consume larger amounts of THC in THCa form
- Layer Therapies!
- Always include a topical application

As a Caregiver

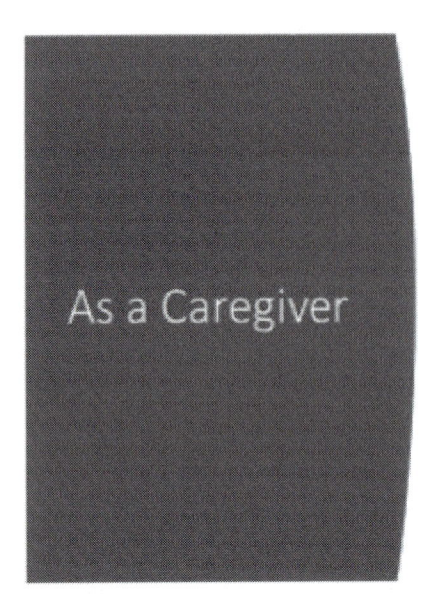

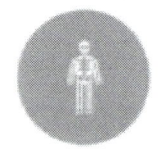

- ASSSURE CANNACIAN GUILDELINES ARE FOLLOWED
- ESTABLISH A CANNABIS ROUTINE
- MONTOR PATIENT CLOSELY
- JOURNAL DAILY

Developing a Therapy Plan

Develop a Therapy Plan with a VERY Slow and Steady approach based on sublingual vs. Edible based doses

Edibles only before bed

Assure patient can be dosed adequately thoughout the day

Know when to add vapor to the routine

Collaborate with other caregivers and Communicate via Journaling

For the Healthy Senior

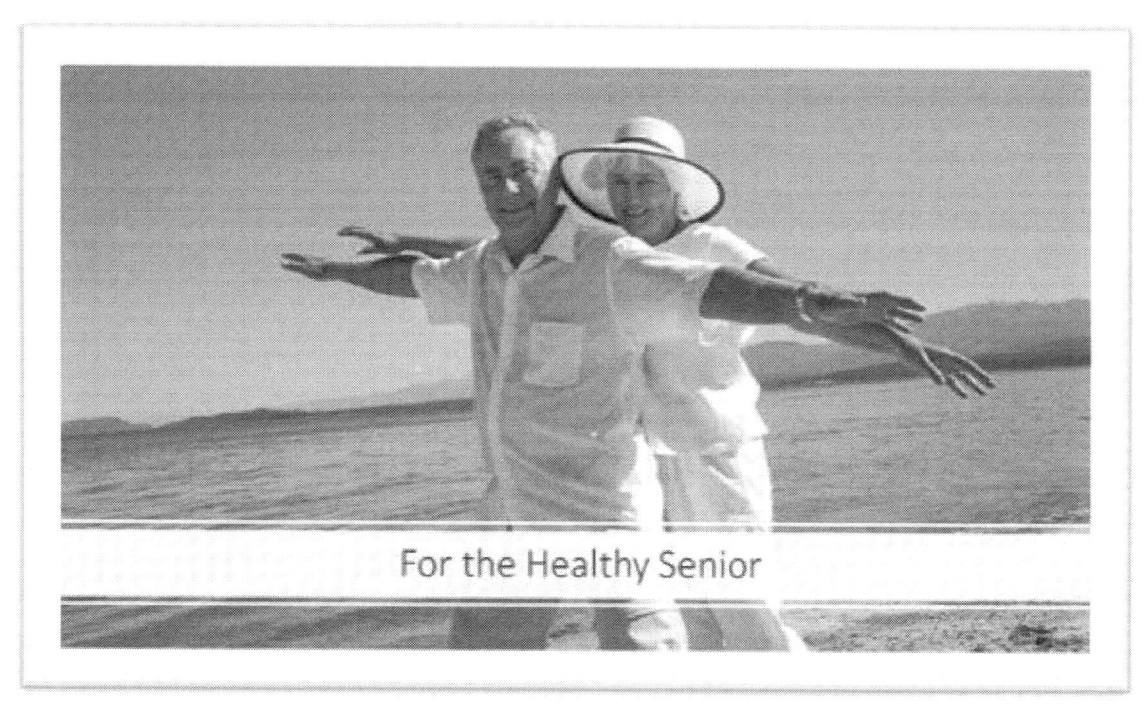

Using cannabis as a daily dietary supplement via hemp oil at 1 mg per kilo minimum dose.

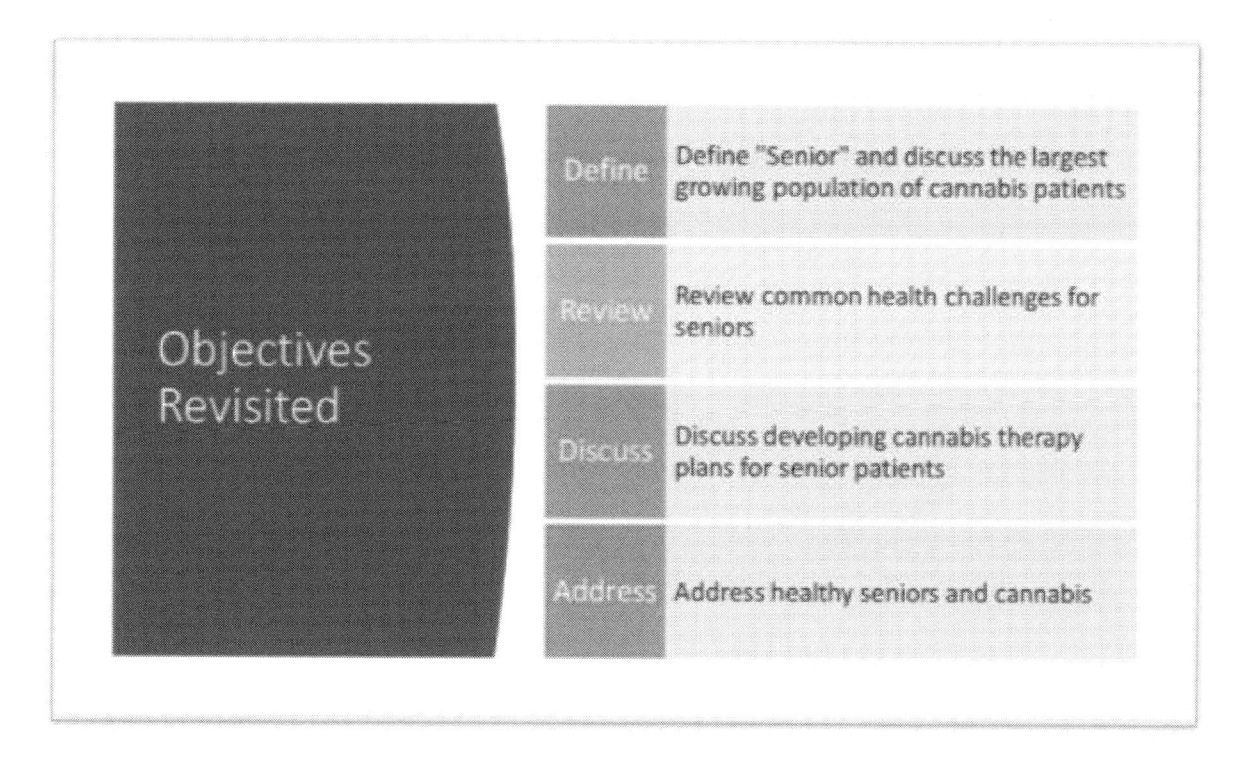

Objectives Revisited

Define	Define "Senior" and discuss the largest growing population of cannabis patients
Review	Review common health challenges for seniors
Discuss	Discuss developing cannabis therapy plans for senior patients
Address	Address healthy seniors and cannabis

Notes

Notes

Notes

Notes

Notes

Notes

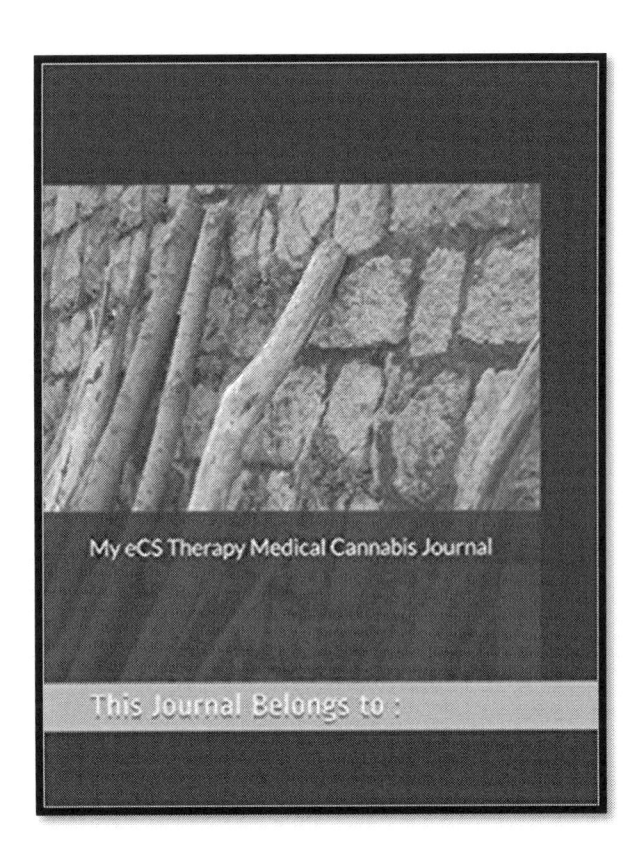

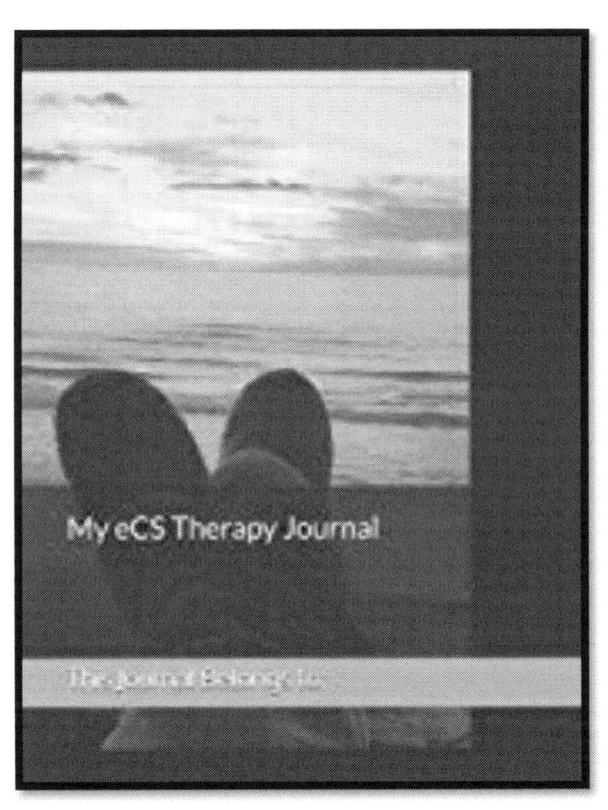

An EASY way to Journal
Get YOURS Today on Amazon
Or at www.MyECSTherapy>org

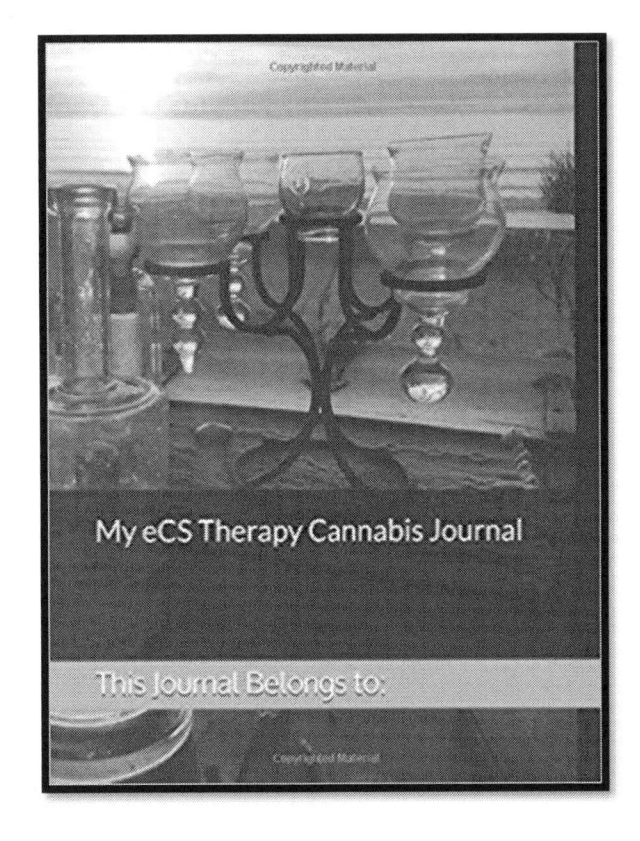

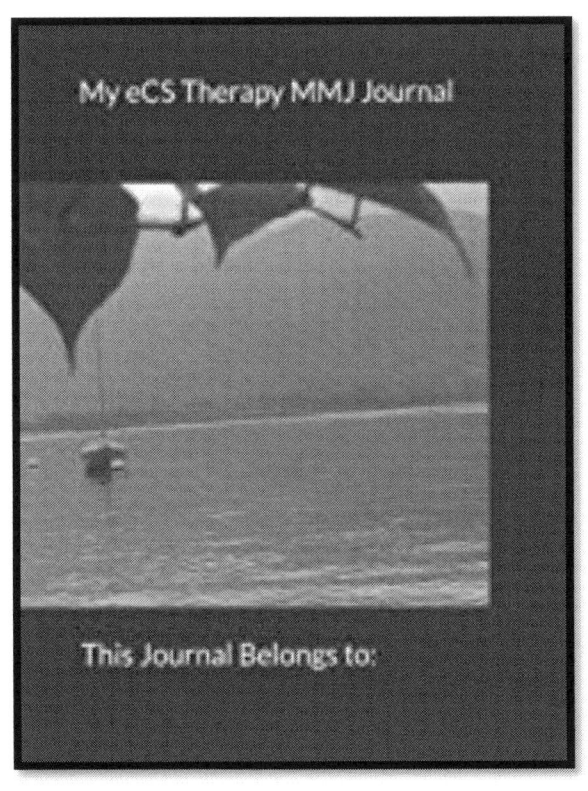

PLANT A SEED FOR CANNABIS EDUCATION TOUR

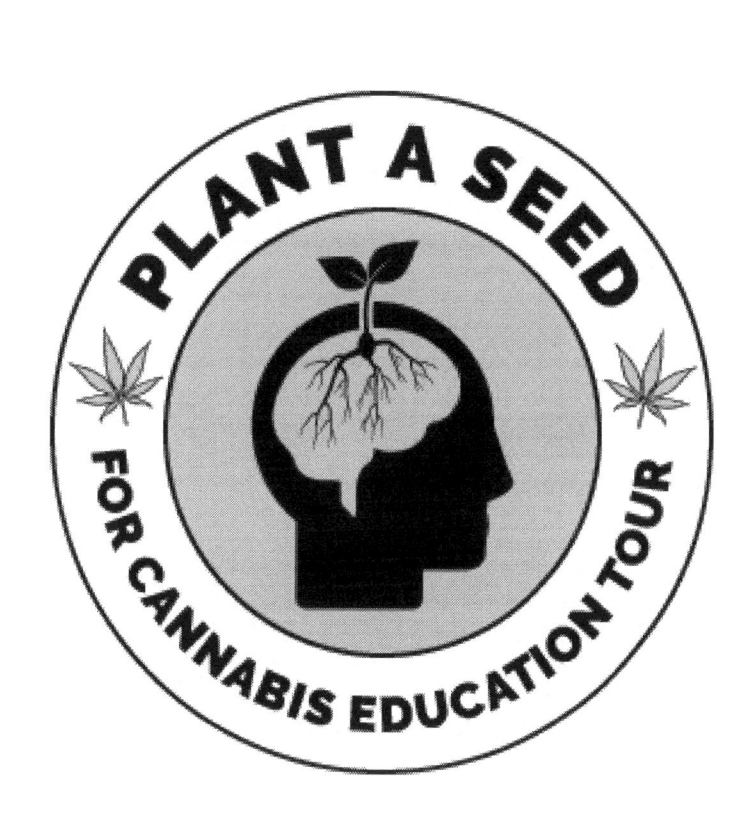

THE SURVIVOR'S GUIDE TO
MEDICAL CANNABIS

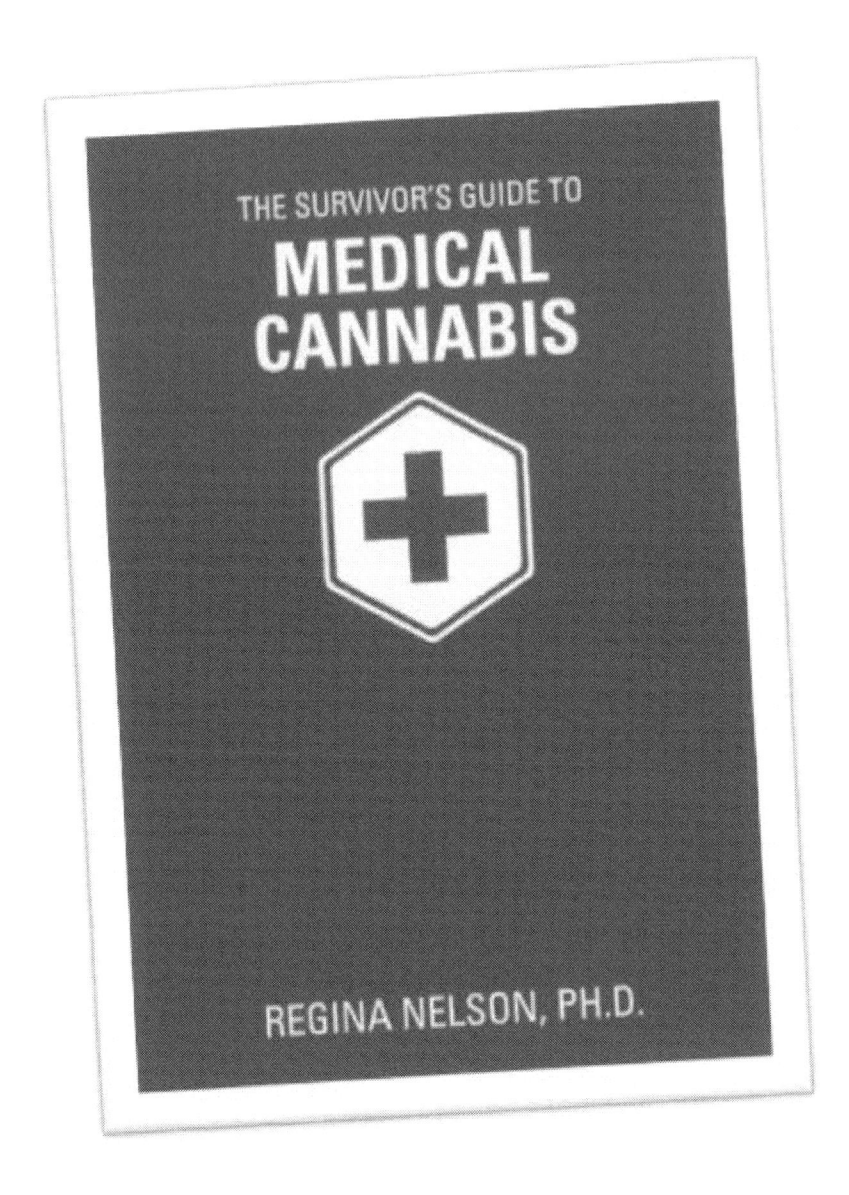

REGINA NELSON, PH.D.

Available at
www.myecstherapy.org

Made in the USA
Middletown, DE
15 November 2021